Rabbits

Health, Husbandry and Diseases

V.C.G. Richardson

MA VetMB MRCVS

b

**Blackwell
Science**

© 2000 by
Blackwell Science Ltd
Editorial Offices:
Osney Mead, Oxford OX2 0EL
25 John Street, London WC1N 2BL
23 Ainslie Place, Edinburgh EH3 6AJ
350 Main Street, Malden
   MA 02148 5018, USA
54 University Street, Carlton
   Victoria 3053, Australia
10, rue Casimir Delavigne
   75006 Paris, France

Other Editorial Offices:

Blackwell Wissenschafts-Verlag GmbH
Kurfürstendamm 57
10707 Berlin, Germany

Blackwell Science KK
MG Kodenmacho Building
7–10 Kodenmacho Nihombashi
Chuo-ku, Tokyo 104, Japan

First published 2000

Set in 10/13.5pt Souvenir
by DP Photosetting, Aylesbury, Bucks
Printed and bound in Great Britain by
MPG Books Ltd, Bodmin, Cornwall

The Blackwell Science logo is a trade mark of
Blackwell Science Ltd, registered at the
United Kingdom Trade Marks Registry

DISTRIBUTORS

Marston Book Services Ltd
PO Box 269
Abingdon
Oxon OX14 4YN
(*Orders:* Tel: 01235 465500
         Fax: 01235 465555)

USA
Blackwell Science, Inc.
Commerce Place
350 Main Street
Malden, MA 02148 5018
(*Orders:* Tel: 800 759 6102
            781 388 8250
         Fax: 781 388 8255)

Canada
Login Brothers Book Company
324 Saulteaux Crescent
Winnipeg, Manitoba R3J 3T2
(*Orders:* Tel: 204 837 2987
         Fax: 204 837 3116)

Australia
Blackwell Science Pty Ltd
54 University Street
Carlton, Victoria 3053
(*Orders:* Tel: 03 9347 0300
         Fax: 03 9347 5001)

A catalogue record for this title is available
from the British Library

ISBN 0-632-05221-X

Library of Congress
Cataloging-in-Publication Data
Rabbits: health, husbandry, and diseases/
   V.C.G. Richardson.
       p. cm.
      Includes bibliographical references
(p.   ).
      ISBN 0-632-05221-X (pbk.)
      1. Rabbits—Diseases. 2. Rabbits—
Health. 3. Rabbits.
I. Richardson, V.C.G.
SF997.5.R2R335   1999
636.9'322—dc21   99-38989
                                  CIP

For further information on
Blackwell Science, visit our website:
www.blackwell-science.com

CONTENTS

PREFACE

The status of the rabbit as a pet has changed dramatically in recent years. For many it is no longer the forgotten pet in a hutch at the bottom of the garden; instead it has been brought indoors and cared for as one of the family, often alongside more traditional family pets, the cat and dog. The 'house rabbit' has become an increasingly popular pet. For working families it may be a dog or cat substitute, as it is happy to be alone all day, but will enjoy and respond to companionship every evening, at a time when it is naturally active. Rabbits are surprisingly responsive and easy to train. The opportunities for free exercise and social contact for the house rabbit create a pet that is often healthier, both physically and emotionally, than its outdoor counterpart.

It is little wonder that our clients now expect, and deserve, the same standard of veterinary care for their rabbits as they receive for their cats and dogs. Previous texts have been concerned, in whole or in part, with laboratory or farmed rabbits. This text, the first of its kind, is devoted entirely to the pet rabbit, its husbandry and health.

As with the treatment of other small pets, the majority of drugs available are not licensed for use in rabbits. Every effort has been made to ensure that the dose rates in the text are accurate, but all drugs must be used at the clinician's own risk. Where appropriate licensed drugs should be selected before non-licensed alternatives.

My thanks go to Fiona Webb and Ean Richardson for providing the photographs used in the book.

V.C.G. Richardson

1 HUSBANDRY

INTRODUCTION

Traditionally, rabbits have been kept as pets in hutches in the garden, in solitary confinement. However, as more has been learnt about the rabbit, and due to alterations in our society, this is all changing. It is now recognised that rabbits are very social creatures, and benefit from company, either from another rabbit, guinea pig, or their owners. They can also interact happily with other pets in the household such as dogs and cats.

The rabbit is the third most popular pet after the dog and cat, and social changes suggest that their popularity is set to increase. With more families working long hours, a dog may become too much of a commitment and cats, being more independent, are often out hunting when their owners are home from work and looking for their companionship. The rabbit is an excellent alternative, as it is able to be shut away in its hutch whilst its owners are at work, yet can offer companionship when they are home. A rabbit is crepuscular by nature, and therefore most active in the morning and evening, when its owners are at home, and naturally content to rest during the day when they are out. Thus there is a growing trend for rabbits to be kept indoors as 'house rabbits'. This chapter reflects these changes, particularly in the sections on housing and stocking.

HOUSING

Rabbits can be kept in a variety of ways, either indoors or outdoors. This may range from a hutch in the garden, shed or garage, to an indoor kennel in the house. Wherever they are kept there are several basic principles that should be considered.

- They should be allowed as much space as possible, with the opportunity for free exercise for 4 hours daily.
- The accommodation should offer one sheltered, dark retreat. This 'den' mimics the burrow and offers a place of safety in which to hide.
- The accommodation should be high enough to allow the rabbit to stand full stretch on its hind legs.
- Rabbits are particularly susceptible to heat stroke; they should not be exposed to direct sunlight in the heat of the day without provision of shade and shelter.

Outdoor rabbits

Many rabbits are kept outdoors in hutches. Ideally there should be a run attached. If the garden is enclosed the rabbit can be allowed free run of the garden. It is important to ensure protection from predators, either wild animals or other domestic pets. The hutch must be situated in a site protected from rain, wind and, in the summer, direct sunlight. Outdoor rabbits must be kept clean and dry and their hutch cleaned regularly, as they are most susceptible to the unwanted attentions of flies and the development of 'fly strike'. Breeders may keep their rabbits in tiers of hutches in a shed or garage. If many rabbits are kept like this it is important to ensure good ventilation at all times. The ideal environmental temperature in a shed is 16°C (61°F). If rabbits are kept in a garage, the car should ideally be kept elsewhere to avoid the effects of noxious car fumes. Rabbits are also particularly terrified of the smell of car oils and petrol.

Indoor rabbits

A variety of accommodation is available for the indoor rabbit. Even if the rabbit is allowed free run of the house, it is important to provide it with a den of its own. The indoor dog kennel is the most popular form of indoor cage. However, as 'house rabbits' become more popular there are 'designer hutches' appearing on the market. It is important that the indoor cage is sited somewhere quiet in the house, and that within the cage there is a dark covered area to hide; the cage should not be placed directly by a radiator or window.

When the rabbit is allowed free run of the house it is important to 'bunny-proof' any electrical wires or other objects that the rabbit may chew.

THE ENVIRONMENT

Rabbits are intelligent creatures that require mental stimulation in order to avoid stereotypical behaviour associated with zoo animals. This is particularly relevant for rabbits kept in confined hutches. Laboratories have recently recognised this need for mental stimulation, and now keep rabbits in groups and provide 'toys'.

The rabbit's natural curiosity and need to burrow can be satisfied by providing pipes to crawl through, and cardboard boxes to chew and hide under. Its foraging instinct can be developed by scattering food and treats all around its environment, so that it can take time to search for food. Plenty of hay for 'grazing' should be supplied at all times. Edible 'toys' such as straw coasters and baskets will provide hours of amusement, as will small plastic toys marketed for cats.

Heat stroke

Rabbits are particularly susceptible to heat stroke, and this is an important factor to consider when planning their environment. They should not be exposed to direct sunlight in the heat of the day without some shade and shelter being provided. Indoor cages should not be placed directly by a radiator or window.

Clinical signs: Respiratory distress, mouth breathing, weakness, depression, incoordination and convulsions. Body temperature more than 40.5°C (105°F).

Treatment: The rabbit should be sprayed with a water spray or immersed in tepid water. Fluids should be given by intravenous or subcutaneous injection. A shock dose of dexamethasone (2 mg/kg) can be given intravenously.

Bedding

Traditionally hay and straw are used as bedding. Hutches can be lined with newspaper or linoleum for ease of cleaning. Indoor rabbits can be kept on newspaper, linoleum or carpet. Hay and straw serve a dual purpose, as bedding and as the basis of the diet, and should be replenished daily. Both indoor and outdoor rabbits can be trained to use a litter tray, and this makes it much easier to keep the environment clean.

Litter training

Rabbits pass their faeces and urine in chosen areas as part of their natural instinct to mark their territory, and it is this trait which makes them easy to litter train. Both indoor and outdoor rabbits can be taught to use a tray in this way. In the case of outdoor rabbits the tray is placed in the area of the hutch where they defaecate; for indoor rabbits the first tray is placed in their indoor kennel, and subsequent trays can be placed around the house. The following principles apply to both indoor and outdoor rabbits.

- Older rabbits are easiest to litter train, particularly if they have been neutered. This is because they have less of an urge to territory mark in multiple sites.
- Loss of litter box habits may occur at sexual maturity, and this can be corrected by neutering. Inappropriate toileting may also be the first symptom of urinary tract disease.
- Rabbits tend to defaecate as they eat, and can be encouraged to use a tray by placing some tasty pieces of food in one corner, or a hay net above the tray.
- If the rabbit takes to sleeping in the tray, a second tray should be provided with straw, or fleece for it to lie in.
- Type of litter. Clay litter should not be used as it can cause gastro-intestinal obstruction if ingested. It has also been well documented that aromatic hydrocarbons from cedar and pine shavings induce liver disease, resulting in elevated liver enzymes, which should return to normal once the litter is removed. The best litter is paper pulp litter or straw which can be ingested safely.

STOCKING

It has recently become clear that rabbits are social animals, and should have companionship. Traditionally rabbits have been kept alone, or with a guinea pig. Two rabbits will form a very close pair-bond, but house rabbits have been known to form close bonds with cats and dogs, despite the fact that both are the rabbit's natural predators.

Rabbits and guinea pigs

There is much written that states that rabbits and guinea pigs should never be kept together. However, there are many rabbits and guinea pigs that do become close companions for their whole lifetime. When considering this issue the following points must be taken into account:

- Rabbits can kick with force, and are capable of breaking the guinea pig's legs or ribs easily. The guinea pig must be given little dens with entrances that only it can get through.
- The rabbit should be neutered, otherwise it could hurt or scare the guinea pig when it tries to mount it.
- Rabbits can harbour *Bordetella*, harmless to the rabbit, but pathogenic for the guinea pig.
- Guinea pigs have a high daily requirement for vitamin C, generally supplied by the provision of large quantities of green food, possibly more than the rabbit is used to.

Rabbit and rabbit

The very best pair-bond is a neutered male and neutered female. Such a pair will remain close for their lifetime. Two neutered does or two neutered bucks may live together, but these pairings are less reliable, and may result in the odd squabble. Same sex pairs are more likely to work if they are introduced to each other when they are young, ideally under 12 weeks of age, or from the same litter. The ideal scenario is the purchase of a male and female from the same litter. The male can be castrated at 14–15 weeks, and the female spayed at 6 months, and they need never be separated. In spacious environments groups of rabbits can live together peaceably.

Pair-bonded rabbits are extremely close, and this should be taken into consideration if one of the pair is ill, or requires hospitalisation. The sick rabbit will recover more quickly, and not lose the will to live if it is kept with its companion, even if this means hospitalising the companion with it. If one member of the pair dies, the remaining rabbit is likely to be able to form another pair-bond easily, as it will crave companionship.

Rabbits and other domestic pets

House rabbits will form close friendships with dogs and cats, traditionally considered to be their predators. Any introductions must be done gradually, and under close supervision. If rabbits do come into contact with dogs or cats, flea control of the dog and cat is extremely important as the flea is the main carrier of mxyomatosis.

Procedure for pairing two rabbits

As previously mentioned the best pair-bond is a neutered male with a neutered female. If only the male is neutered, the female may experience cycles of moodiness associated with her hormonal surges and the development of false pregnancies, and may become aggressive towards her companion at certain times in this cycle.

- The two rabbits should be introduced on neutral territory, with plenty of available space.
- There will be chasing and mounting by the two rabbits, this is a sexual ritual (even if neutered) and quite normal.
- Only intervene if actual fighting occurs, and then try aversion tactics using a water spray, before handling the rabbits.
- Some rabbits may accept each other almost immediately, but it may take 24–48 hours.
- When the rabbits groom each other, particularly around the head, bonding has been successful.
- Opposite sex rabbits, if neutered, can be paired at any time of the year. Same sex rabbits are best paired in the winter during their period of sexual inactivity, when they are least likely to fight. Same sex pairs should not be able to smell an opposite sex rabbit in their surroundings, or they will fight.
- If a neutered buck is paired with an unneutered doe it must be done at least 2 weeks after the surgery as he could still be able to mate her. The exception is if the doe has not reached sexual maturity, in which instance they can be paired immediately.

2 NUTRITION

The principal components of the rabbit diet are fibre, protein, carbohydrate, vitamins and minerals. Of these fibre is the most important.

FIBRE

Fibre is the single most important component of the rabbit diet. The particle size and digestibility of the fibre are also important.

- The rabbit needs large indigestible fibre particles (containing lignocellulose) to drive the gastrointestinal system, and to maintain healthy peristalsis. Gastric stasis and the subsequent accumulation of a 'felt' of ingesta and hair is rarely seen in rabbits on high fibre diets.
- Large fibre particles ensure the natural wear of the molar teeth with a side-to-side chewing action. Small particles tend to be eaten with a crushing action which encourages unnatural wear on the teeth.
- High fibre, low energy diets will result in complete caecotrophy, and avoid the development of 'sticky bottom syndrome'. Such diets also prevent obesity.
- High fibre (hay) diets allow the rabbit to 'graze' for several hours daily, which closely parallels the behaviour of wild rabbits, and reduces boredom and stress. This reduces fur chewing of itself or its companions, and reduces destructive chewing of the environment.

Fibre should make up 18–20% of the diet, and of this at least 10% should be crude indigestible fibre. As most complementary dry foods contain less than this (between 5.7 and 14%) every diet should be complemented with good hay. Fibre is particularly important for the maintenance of a healthy digestive system: a high fibre diet keeps the correct balance of bacterial flora in the caecum. If the fibre content of the diet falls, the caecal pH alters, and the populations of *Clostridia* and *Escherichia coli* rise. This is particularly significant at lifestages when the gastrointestinal system is most vulnerable, such as weaning, or during antibiotic usage. Rabbits on high fibre diets rarely suffer from mucoid enteritis, or enterotoxaemia. High fibre diets will also protect against enterotoxaemia when antibiotics are given.

PROTEIN

The recommended protein level of the diet is 12–13%. Higher protein levels of 17–18% may be used for breeding stock, and 15% for growth. Protein is part of the concentrated ration, but is also found in hay.

High protein diets will lead to an increase in the production and excretion of ammonia, and this may increase the rabbit's susceptibility to respiratory disorders, and eye infections. Excess protein may also lead to incomplete coprophagy and the development of 'sticky bottom syndrome'.

FAT

The dietary requirement for fat is 1–3%; 1% fat is suitable for maintenance, and 3% for pregnancy and growth. However, many rations have increased fat content to increase palatability. The fat content of concentrated food is listed in the food analysis as oil. Vegetable oils, soya and linseed are more digestible than animal fats.

Excess dietary fat may lead to the development of arteriosclerosis. A fat deficiency is rare; however, the oils in the dry food are the rabbit's only source of essential fatty acids, and if the dry food that is fed is old or musty, an essential fatty acid deficiency will manifest as a dry dull haircoat.

CARBOHYDRATE

Rabbits have little requirement for carbohydrate. However, many pet and house rabbits are fed starchy and sugary treats regularly. This causes obesity and encourages enterotoxaemia. The 'starch overload' theory suggests that excess carbohydrates will exceed the stomach's capacity to absorb them, and these carbohydrates provide fuel in the caecum for the multiplication of *E. coli* and *Clostridia*.

VITAMINS AND MINERALS

During the process of digestion the microflora in the caecum synthesise vitamins B, C and K. These are then returned to the rabbit in the caeco-trophes ingested during caecotrophy. Vitamins A, D and E are included in the pelleted ration. Concentrated ration should not be stored for longer than 3 months as the vitamin content will deteriorate over time.

Vitamin B and K supplementation must be considered for rabbits that are unable to practise caecotrophy.

Vitamin A

This should be incorporated into the average concentrate ration at a rate of 10 000 iu/kg. Vitamin A deficiency will result in infertility, abortions, resorption and increased neonatal mortality. Vitamin A deficiency or excess can cause hydrocephalus. Alfalfa is rich in vitamin A, and if fed alongside vitamin A rich pellets may also lead to the development of hydrocephalus.

Hepatic coccidiosis will lower the liver levels of both vitamins A and E.

Vitamin C

This vitamin is also synthesised during the process of digestion. However vitamin C supplementation may be of benefit in the treatment of respira-tory disease, and in the prevention of enterotoxaemia, as it may inhibit toxin production. It can be given at a dose of 50–100 mg/kg daily. Overdosage does not occur as any excess is excreted through the kidneys.

Vitamin D

This is incorporated into the average concentrate ration at a rate of 900 iu/kg. Excess vitamin D may be a factor in excessive calcium uptake, and the development of dystrophic calcification of renal and aortic blood vessels (at levels of 2300 iu/kg of feed) although the rabbit has a unique calcium metabolism (see calcium).

Vitamin E

This is incorporated into the average concentrate ration at a rate of 50 mg/kg. Vitamin E deficiency can lead to reduced fertility, and additional vitamin E can be added to the diet by supplementation with wheatgerm. Vitamin E deficiency can cause muscular dystrophy and hind leg paralysis in young rabbits. These symptoms may be seen if less than 16 mg/kg vitamin E is incorporated into the diet. Blood biochemistry in a case of hypovitaminosis E will reveal a raised creatine phosphokinase (CPK).

Calcium

The rabbit has an unusual calcium metabolism. The level of plasma calcium is not regulated by vitamin D and parathyroid hormone as in other mammals, but varies directly with the level of dietary calcium. Excess calcium is excreted through the urinary system, making bladder and kidney stones a common occurrence if diets are high in calcium. Metastatic calcification can also occur with high calcium diets. Conversely, as much of the dietary calcium is held in the pelleted portion of the ration, rabbits that are selective feeders and leave their pellets may have a low calcium intake. This leads to osteoporosis, particularly evident in the vertebrae, and jaw bones. Poor mineralisation of the teeth, and acquired malocclusion are consequences of a diet too low in calcium. Osteoporosis of the vertebrae leads to vertebral fractures.

The daily requirement for calcium of a medium-sized pet rabbit is approximately 510 mg.

Copper

Copper is added in the form of cupric sulphate to the concentrate ration at a rate of 4–30 mg/kg. It is thought to reduce enteritis and increase weight gain in young stock. There are no toxic effects from feeding this level of copper.

RECOMMENDED DIET

The basic pet rabbit diet should consist of hay, greens and a dry mix (concentrate). Fibre in the form of hay is the single most important part of any diet. Rabbits fed on a basic hay and greens diet are unlikely to suffer from obesity, digestive problems, or 'sticky bottom syndrome' (chronic excess caecal pellets). Water is a necessity, and treats may also be given sparingly.

Hay

Various types of hay are available, grass hay, clover hays, and alfalfa. Grass hay is best, as it is lower in calories and calcium than alfalfa. Some dry mixes contain alfalfa, and if alfalfa hay is also fed the diet is likely to contain excess calcium. Chopped dried grass ('Readygrass') formulated for horses can be given. Such grass is of a consistent quality, and is not dusty, in comparison with some forms of grass hay. The protein content varies with the type of hay fed, and this will affect the total protein levels of a diet when combining hay with dry rations.

Hay type	Protein	Fibre	Calcium
Alfalfa	16%	28%	1.5%
Grass hay	14%	31%	0.4%
Timothy	8%	30%	0.5%
Wheat straw	3%	35%	0.2%

Fresh greens

A wide variety of greens, both cultivated and wild, can be included in the diet. If a rabbit is unused to greens they should be introduced slowly, and any that cause diarrhoea should be withdrawn. Eventually greens can be given ad libitum. Wild plants are particularly useful, as most are astringent and have medical properties. Any plants should be collected away from contamination of car exhaust or dog urine, and washed before feeding.

Concentrate ration

Various rabbit pellets and 'complementary' dry foods are available. They are the least important part of the diet and should be given as an adjunct to the hay and greens diet. The fibre content of all dry foods falls short of the daily requirement and the extra fibre will be provided by the hay and greens. Some contain alfalfa or alfalfa pellets, and these rations are higher in calcium. Rabbits that eat too much dry food have a tendency towards obesity and gastrointestinal disturbances. Some rabbits may selectively pick out components of the mix and leave the pellets, and consequently receive a diet that is too low in calcium and develop osteoporosis. Burgess SupaRabbit Excel is formulated as extruded nuggets and each nugget is nutritionally balanced to avoid the problem of selective feeding.

The dry food should be fed in small quantities to complement the hay and greens diet, and the rabbit should be encouraged to eat the whole ration before the bowl is refilled.

Treats

There are many proprietary treat foods on the pet market, and owners of house rabbits are likely to give them sugary and carbohydrate-rich foods such as biscuits and cakes. Rabbits, like children, can become junk-food addicts, and selectively choose the sugary, starchy foods that are bad for them. This practice leads to obesity and an increased risk of gastro-intestinal disturbance, as the overload of carbohydrate and sugar in the caecum allows harmful bacteria to multiply. Dental caries can also develop.

The replacement of sugary treats with fruit should be encouraged. Rabbits can be given wicker baskets, or placemats as 'edible toys'. The occasional dry breakfast cereal such as Shredded Wheat with no added salt or sugar, or a slice of brown toast is acceptable, but rabbits should be given these infrequently.

Water

Fresh water should be available at all times, even when the rabbit eats a large amount of greens and may seemingly not drink much. Water can be provided in bowls or sipper bottles; the latter is more hygienic. It is important to use whichever the rabbit is familiar with, as if presented with an unfamiliar water source the rabbit may fail to drink, and dehydrate. Sipper bottles must be cleaned regularly, and checked for leakage. 'Blue fur disease' is a moist dermatitis associated with *Pseudomonas* contamination of leaking sipper bottles.

EDIBLE WILD PLANTS

The feeding of wild plants can help provide a varied and interesting diet, as well as reduce feeding costs. Plants should be collected from areas not contaminated by dogs or pollution, or from fields sprayed with chemicals. All plants should be washed before feeding.

Many of the plants have medicinal properties, and these are detailed below.

- Agrimony – astringent, tonic and a diuretic
- Avens – astringent

- Bramble – astringent
- Chickweed
- Clover – good source of protein. Tonic, useful during moult
- Coltsfoot – good for respiratory disorders
- Cow parsnip (hogweed) – useful for nursing does
- Dandelion – laxative and diuretic
- Goosegrass – diuretic, tonic
- Ground elder – feed leaves only before it flowers
- Groundsel – laxative. Tonic, useful during moult
- Knapweed – astringent
- Mallow – astringent. Expectorant, useful for respiratory disorders
- Mayweed
- Plantain – astringent, diuretic and antimicrobial
- Raspberry – leaves are astringent. Has an action on the uterine muscle making parturition easier
- Sea beet
- Shepherd's purse – astringent and tonic
- Sow thistle – useful for lactating does
- Trefoil
- Vetch
- Wild strawberry – astringent
- Yarrow – astringent, diuretic and a urinary antiseptic

Grass

Grass is one of the most neglected components of the rabbit diet. Whilst its wild counterparts feed exclusively on grass, most pet rabbits are never given fresh grass, although they receive dried grass as hay. Grass is an excellent source of fibre and has a more abrasive action on the teeth than hay. Eating grass encourages the side-to-side chewing action essential for the proper wear of the molars. Grass should be gradually introduced into the diet, particularly in the spring when the grass growth is rapid, as eating too much at this time can cause digestive upsets. The grass that is fed should be pulled rather than as grass clippings as the latter have a tendency to overheat and ferment, again causing digestive disturbances.

EDIBLE CULTIVATED PLANTS

A large selection of vegetables and fruits can be fed. They are detailed here in groups according to their calcium content, as this can be important when using vegetables to correct urinary disorders, or to prevent osteoporosis.

Good calcium sources

- Chinese cabbage
- Watercress
- Kale
- Dandelions
- Parsley
- Spinach

Moderate calcium sources

- Cabbage
- Strawberries
- Radish and radish tops

Poor calcium sources

- Carrots*
- Cauliflower
- Celery
- Cucumber
- Lettuce
- Tomato*
- Bananas*
- Brussels sprouts
- Apples

Those marked with an asterisk should not be fed to rabbits with renal dysfunction due to their high phosphorus content.

FEEDING REGIMES FOR LIFESTAGES

Weaning

For the first 21 days of its life the young rabbit is totally dependent on its mother's milk. At 3 weeks of age it will begin to nibble at foods, and by 6–8 weeks it will be independent of its mother, and eating all solid food. It is during this transition period that it is very vulnerable to developing gastrointestinal disorders, notably enterotoxaemia.

It is extremely important that there is plenty of good quality hay available for the young rabbit as soon as it begins to nibble at solid food. The young rabbits will inevitably start eating their mother's dry food, but care must be taken not to overfeed them with the concentrated ration, as the risk of developing caecal dysbiosis is increased as the energy content of the diet increases. Any adjustment to their diet should be done slowly, each change being made over a 5 day period.

A probiotic can be added to the drinking water over this period of weaning, to give added protection against the development of enterotoxaemia.

Growth

A ration with up to 18% protein can be given to growing rabbits. There must be plenty of good quality hay available, as increasing the protein content can increase the risk of caecal dysbiosis. A varied selection of green foods should be offered on a daily basis. At this stage a ration containing alfalfa will ensure that the calcium intake is sufficient for the development of strong bones.

Breeding

Breeding rabbits and nursing does should receive a ration of 18% protein and 18–20% fibre. The ration can contain alfalfa to ensure that the lactating doe does not develop hypocalcaemia and osteoporosis. Breeding rabbits must be fit and in good condition. Obese animals may fail to breed, and these should be put on a 2–3 week hay-only diet, and then the concentrate ration reintroduced. They should be mated when they are on this rising plane of nutrition. Wheatgerm oil (a good source of vitamin E) can be given on the food at a rate of a few drops daily to breeding stock to improve fertility.

The adult pet

Many adult rabbits have a tendency towards obesity, particularly hutch rabbits with little opportunity for exercise. House rabbits with free run of the house are generally fitter and can be fed accordingly. The pet rabbit should receive plenty of hay, fresh greens, and a limited amount of concentrate mix. Obese hutch rabbits can live on hay and greens alone. It must be ensured that house rabbits receive plenty of hay; it is sometimes left out of the diet as it is considered messy indoors. Alfalfa is too high in calcium and protein for these rabbits. A diet of 13% protein and 18–20% fibre is sufficient for maintenance.

POISONOUS PLANTS

Although it is often assumed that rabbits can instinctively tell which plants are edible and which ones are not, this is not always the case; as rabbits are unable to vomit the ingestion of poisonous plants can be fatal.

The following lists are important if rabbits are allowed free grazing in the garden, or if wild plants are picked for fodder. These are not exhaustive lists, but cover the most commonly encountered plants, with notes on treatment where applicable.

Poisonous wild plants

- All plants that grow from bulbs (crocus, bluebell, etc.)
- Anemones
- Arum ('lords and ladies')
- Bracken
- Bryony
- Buttercup (although this is safe if small quantities are found dried in hay)
- Celandine
- Charlock
- Convolvulus (bindweed)
- Deadly nightshade (belladonna)
- Docks once the flowers appear as the woody leaves contain oxalic acid which causes renal failure
- Figwort
- Flags (*Iris* spp.)
- Fool's parsley
- Foxglove – this contains digitalis, a heart stimulant, and symptoms include tremor and fitting. The symptoms may be controlled by administering oral calcium in the liquid form; for example, Collo-cal D (C-Vet), which contains 0.75% w/v colloidal calcium oleate and 70 iu/ml vitamin D, may be given at a dose of 0.5 ml/kg twice daily.

- Ground elder once the flowers appear, as its action then becomes too diuretic
- Hellebore
- Hemlock
- Henbane
- Horsetails
- Iris
- Lily of the valley
- Monkshood
- Oak leaves – these will cause renal failure
- Poppies
- Privet
- Ragwort – this causes fatal liver failure
- Scarlet pimpernel
- Speedwell
- Spurge
- Toadflax ('old man's beard')
- Travellers joy
- Wild celery

Poisonous cultivated plants

- All plants grown from bulbs (crocus, daffodils, lilies, etc.)
- Castor oil plant
- Cloth of gold
- Datura
- Horse chestnut
- Juniper trees
- Laburnum
- Laurels
- Lupins
- Morning glory
- Nightshades
- Pokeweed
- Primroses (*Primula* spp.)
- Privet
- Rhododendron
- Solomon's seal
- Spindle trees

- Star of Bethlehem
- Sumach trees
- Yew
- Wisteria.

3 THE CLINICAL EXAMINATION

Before the examination it is important to obtain a full history of the patient. First the age, sex (neutered?) and the clinical complaint should be recorded. Details of husbandry and diet are essential; whether the rabbit is an outdoor or house rabbit, whether it lives alone, or with other rabbits or guinea pigs. When considering its diet, does it get treats, does it eat all its complete food or just select its favourite pieces, does it have access to plants in its environment, whether house or garden? Because many conditions are associated with poor husbandry and nutritional imbalances, it is important to make these investigations as comprehensive as possible.

Once the history has been taken, the rabbit should be observed in its box or carrier before it is handled. The speed and depth of respiration should be noted: rabbits are obligate nose breathers and mouth breathing is a poor prognostic sign. The normal respiratory rate is 30–60 breaths/minute, and slow, deep respiration is abnormal. The rabbit should look comfortable and alert, the eyes should be bright and the nose should twitch regularly. The presence of a head tilt or nystagmus will be evident at this time.

A rabbit that is in pain will sit in a hunched position, and may grind its teeth loudly.

HANDLING

Rabbits must be handled very carefully. Although they are generally docile they are apt to struggle when picked up, with potentially harmful consequences. All rabbits are prone to vertebral fractures, and this risk is greatest in hutch rabbits or in those on an unbalanced diet that may have concurrent osteoporosis. It is extremely important to support the back and hindquarters whenever a rabbit is handled.

A rabbit should never be picked up by the ears. It can be lifted gently by the scruff of the neck with one hand whilst the other hand supports its bottom (Figure 3.1), or alternatively lifted with one hand under the chest, and one supporting its hindquarters (Figure 3.2). The rabbit should be carried against the body to minimise struggling. It is advisable to place the rabbit's carrying box on the floor so that if it does jump as it is picked up it does not hurt itself. Similarly it is usually easier to return the rabbit to the box on the floor at the end of the examination.

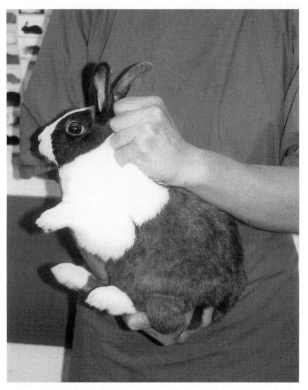

Figure 3.1   Rabbit being held correctly with one hand holding scruff of neck while the other hand supports the hindquarters.

The rabbit should be placed on a non-slip surface for the examination. It should be restrained with a hand on its scruff all the time. Some rabbits are calmed if their eyes are covered with the other hand. The majority of the examination can be done in this position; however, it may be easier to hold the rabbit on its back to examine its incisors, and to trim toenails. For this the assistant holds the rabbit against their body with its back supported with one arm, and the hand steadying the outside hind leg. The other hand is cupped over the chest (Figure 3.3). Alternatively the rabbit can be held by

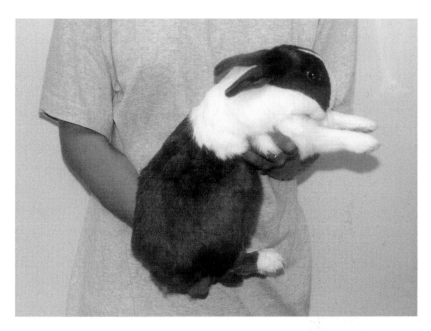

Figure 3.2 An alternative way of correctly holding a rabbit is to place one hand under the chest and support the hindquarters with the other hand.

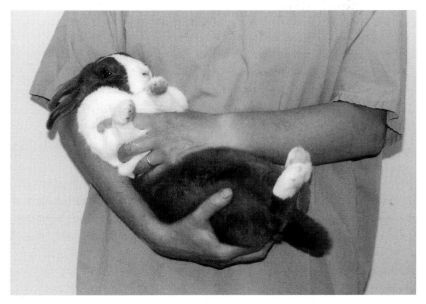

Figure 3.3 Rabbits can also be held with their back supported by one arm and one hand steadying the outside hind leg, with the second hand cupped over the chest.

the scruff with the left hand and the back supported by the left arm (Figure 3.4). This frees the other hand for other procedures. Rabbits can be kept calm in this position, and if the handler gently strokes the bridge of the nose whilst talking gently they can be 'tranced' (hypnotised) (Figure 3.5). Their heart rate and respiration rate do not increase in this position, indicating that they do not find it stressful.

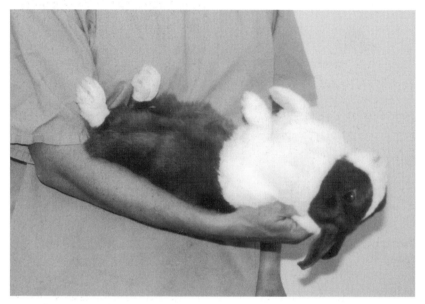

Figure 3.4   The rabbit can be held by the scruff of the neck with one hand, and with the back supported by the other arm.

For palpation of the abdomen it may be easiest to hold the rabbit vertically, with its back against the handler's body, and one hand supporting the chest (Figure 3.6). This frees the other hand to examine the rabbit.

If a rabbit is too fractious or nervous to examine, it may be necessary to sedate it so that the examination can be carried out without injury. Diazepam can be given at a dose of 1–2 mg/kg by intramuscular injection.

THE EXAMINATION

The examination should be conducted in a logical manner so that each system is investigated. Beginning at the head, the incisors should be

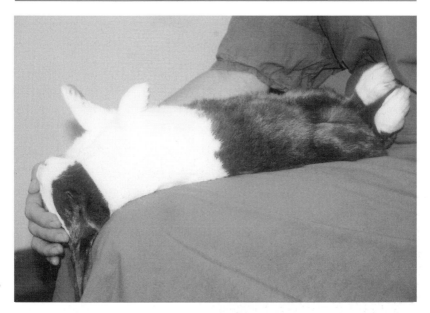

Figure 3.5 Rabbits can be tranced if the handler gently strokes the bridge of the nose while talking gently.

inspected for enamel quality and signs of malocclusion. The molars are harder to inspect: an aural or vaginal speculum will help visualise these back teeth; however, if dental problems are suspected a fuller examination will be required under sedation, as it is possible to miss lesions with a speculum. A wet chin, or dampness on the medial aspect of the forelegs will indicate that the rabbit has been dribbling through dental discomfort. The lower jaw should be felt for any bony abnormalities, or abscesses that may be associated with the tooth roots.

The head should be held level, and the eyes should be examined for even pupil size and other ocular abnormalities. There should be no ocular discharge, and pressure at the medial canthus of the eye will reveal any purulent material in the tear duct. The nares should be examined for the presence of a nasal discharge, and again the medial aspect of the forelegs may be matted with discharge as the rabbit wipes its nose. The ears should be examined for the presence of exudate. Normal ear wax is golden in colour, but a dry crusty exudate is seen with ear mites.

The thorax should be auscultated. Interpretation of chest sounds requires experience, as referred upper airway sounds are normal because the rabbit breaths through its nose. Many rabbits also have a degree of dry, adventitious noise associated with previous low grade respiratory infections. The

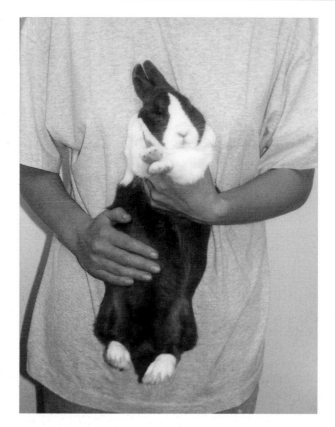

Figure 3.6 For palpation of the abdomen, it is easier to hold the rabbit vertically with its back against the handler's body, and one hand supporting the chest.

heart rate is usually 120–250 beats/minute. Rabbits in severe respiratory distress will have an arrhythmic heart rate (above 200 beats/minute) and cyanosed mucous membranes. Abdominal pain may present as respiratory distress.

The abdomen should be palpated gently because the organs can bruise and haemorrhage easily. The presence of gastric bloat, gastric ileus and caecal ileus can be detected on examination. The abdomen can also be auscultated for the presence of gut sounds: an absence of sounds will indicate ileus.

Abnormalities of the uterus such as uterine adenocarcinoma may be palpable. The presence of growths or cysts in the mammary tissue may indicate this as a likely diagnosis. The bladder should be palpated very gently, as it is thin-walled and easily ruptured. Further investigation of the bladder and other abdominal organs may require radiography. The kidneys may be easiest to palpate with the rabbit in dorsal recumbency: the left kidney is very mobile.

The limbs should be examined for abnormalities. The plantar aspect of the hocks is a frequent site of inflammation and haemorrhage (podo-dermatitis). Rabbits that are presented because the owner has found some blood in the cage should have their toenails and hocks examined carefully, together with the routine genitourinary investigation.

Examination of the skin includes a search for wounds, abscesses and mite infestations. The perineal area and dorsum should be examined closely for blowfly myiasis, especially in any rabbit that is 'off colour' in warm humid weather.

The rabbit should be weighed. This is particularly important if any medication is to be administered. Paediatric scales are ideal for this purpose (Figure 3.7).

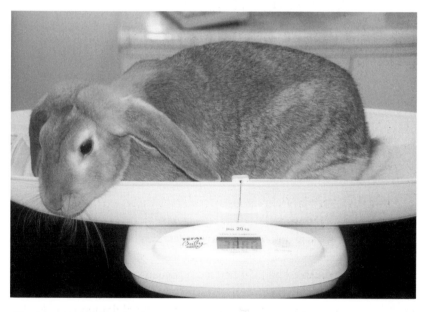

Figure 3.7 Paediatric scales are ideal for weighing rabbits.

The rectal temperature can be taken at the clinician's own judgement, as the findings are often not helpful in making a diagnosis. The normal rabbit temperature is 38.5–40°C (101.3–104°F); however, this can increase with stress or during a period in a carrier in the waiting room. Conversely sick animals generally have a low body temperature.

DIAGNOSTIC PROCEDURES

The most readily available procedures for further diagnosis are radiography and blood testing. Radiography is performed as in other companion animals, and its interpretation is discussed where appropriate throughout this text. Ultrasound, if available, is also a useful diagnostic tool.

As with radiography, some chemical restraint may be necessary to facilitate blood sampling. Blood samples can be collected from the cephalic vein, the lateral saphenous vein, or the jugular vein. The marginal ear vein or the central auricular artery can also be used for small samples, although these may carry an increased risk of thrombosis and skin sloughing. The jugular vein is a useful site if a larger amount of blood is needed (2–3 ml). The rabbit can be held in sternal or dorsal recumbency with the neck extended, and the jugular vein is evident running from the thoracic inlet to the base of the ear. This vein may be difficult to access in does with a large dewlap.

Interpretation of results

The majority of research done on haematology and biochemistry has been performed on laboratory animals, and often a wide range of normal values are recorded in the literature. The majority of clinical laboratories will have their own list of normal values, and these are often the most useful guideline when interpreting the results.

Haematology

The rabbit has a few peculiarities which are worth a mention. Rabbit neutrophils (known as heterophils) have brilliant eosinophilic granules, and look more like eosinophils. The nucleus of the neutrophil is usually visible. Eosinophils are larger, and their bilobed nucleus may be obscured by large cytoplasmic granules. Basophils are common in normal rabbit blood smears.

The erythrocytes of a rabbit have a life span of 57 days. In a healthy rabbit 2–4% of these erythrocytes may be identified as reticulocytes. 1–2% of the red cells may show a normal anocytosis and polychromasia. The PCV (haematocrit) of a healthy rabbit is between 30 and 50%. Sick rabbits have a tendency to develop anaemia.

The white blood cell count ranges from 3.1×10^9 to 12×10^9 cells/ litre. In a normal rabbit the differential is approximately 30% neutrophils (heterophils) and 60% lymphocytes. Bacterial infections are not often accompanied by a raised white cell count; instead a leucopaenia is more common. Stress may cause a lymphopaenia, eosinopaenia and neutrophilia.

Biochemistry

Some of the biochemical parameters can be affected by restraint, and it is important to ensure that blood sampling is done with the rabbit as calm as possible. In particular the muscle enzymes lactate dehydrogenase (LDH), aspartate aminotransferase (AST) and creatine kinase (CK) will be elevated if the rabbit struggles whilst it is restrained.

Alanine aminotransferase (ALT): 22–80 iu/litre

This enzyme is found in the liver and heart. ALT will be raised in association with liver damage, necrosis and advanced neoplasia.

Alkaline phosphatase (ALKP): 15–90 iu/litre

This enzyme is present in many tissues, associated with the cell membranes. It will increase in any case of tissue inflammation. The highest levels are found in the intestines, liver, osteoblasts and placenta. It will be elevated in young rabbits, liver disease and bone disease. It is reduced in diarrhoea, and during pregnancy.

Aspartate aminotransferase (AST): 14–113 iu/litre

This enzyme is present predominately in liver and muscle. It is also present in the heart, kidney and pancreas. AST will be raised in association with liver damage and *Eimeria stiedae* infection. It will also be elevated if the rabbit struggles during restraint.

Creatine kinase (CK): 50–250 iu/litre

This enzyme is specific to muscle, and will rise rapidly following muscle degeneration. The figure will return relatively quickly to normal once the damage is over. It will rise during a stressful restraint.

γ-*Glutamyltransferase (GGT): 0–7 iu/litre*

This enzyme is found in the kidney and liver. The main source of plasma GGT is the bile duct epithelium, and a raised GGT may indicate post-hepatic biliary obstruction. The enzyme does not increase in cases of hepatocellular necrosis.

Lactate dehydrogenase (LDH): 34–129 iu/litre

This enzyme is present in most cells of the body, and in erythrocytes. It will be elevated during restraint, and also in cases where haemolysis occurs.

Total protein: 54–75 g/litre

Albumin makes up 60% of the total serum protein, and globulin makes up 40%. Albumin, and consequently total protein, will decrease in renal and liver disease. Total proteins will increase with dehydration and shock. They will also increase in heat stroke.

Glucose: 4.2–8.3 mmol/litre

Blood glucose will be elevated during stress, shock and excitement. Diabetes mellitus is very rare in the rabbit.

Calcium: 5.6–12.5 mg/dl (1.39–3.11 mmol/litre)

The rabbit has a unique calcium metabolism, and serum calcium is directly proportional to the calcium in the diet. Low serum calcium will lead to osteoporosis and dental disorders, whilst high serum calcium will result in the formation of urinary calculi.

Blood urea nitrogen (BUN): 17–24 mg/dl (6.06–8.56 mmol/litre)

BUN will increase when 50–70% of renal function is lost, and in cases of renal neoplasia. The BUN will be reduced by low protein diets, the use of anabolic steroids and in severe hepatic insufficiency.

Creatinine: 44–177 mmol/litre

This will increase when 50–70% of renal function is lost.

4 THE SKIN

FUNGAL AND YEAST INFECTIONS

Ringworm

This is caused by the dermatophytes *Trichophyton mentagrophytes* and *Microsporum canis*. *Trichophyton* is more commonly found on outdoor rabbits whilst *Microsporum* is found on house rabbits. It is a zoonosis, and rabbits can serve as a reservoir for human infection.

Clinical signs: Dry scaly lesions initially on the nose and muzzle. The lesions may spread across the face, round the base of the ears and to the feet. The lesions are generally pruritic.

Infection of young rabbits occurs in the nest box, which may become contaminated with the fungal spores. During nursing the young are in direct contact with the skin and fur around the teats, and it is easily transferred to their mouth and muzzle.

Diagnosis: Only *Microsporum* will fluoresce under ultraviolet light (Wood's lamp). Diagnosis is by microscopy and culture on Sabouraud's medium.

Treatment: Griseofulvin given orally at a dose of 25 mg/kg twice daily for 4–6 weeks is effective. The tablets can be broken and given in a little strawberry jam. Griseofulvin should not be given during pregnancy as it is teratogenic.

Washes that can be used in conjunction with griseofulvin include povidone–iodine (Tamodine, Vetark Professional), 1% triclosan (Sporal-D, MediChem International), and enilconazole (Imaverol, Janssen UK Ltd.) at a 1:10 dilution.

Clotrimazole cream can be used topically.

The environment should be thoroughly disinfected. If a shed or building needs to be treated, a solution of enilconazole can be made into a spray and used at a rate of $50\,mg/m^2$ twice weekly for 5 months. Steps should be made to eliminate wild rats and mice from the environment as these are often carriers of the disease.

Candidiasis

Clinical signs: A moist dermatitis, especially under the chin and dewlap, caused by the yeast *Candida albicans*.

Diagnosis: Microscopy of skin scrapings.

Treatment: The area should be bathed daily with 1% chlorhexidine. Daily application of chlorhexidine in aqueous cream, or daily application of an antimycotic should clear the condition in 10–14 days. Natamycin (Myco-phyt, Intervet UK Ltd.) or enilconazole (Imaverol, Janssen, UK Ltd.) used at a 1:50 dilution are suitable.

ECTOPARASITES

Fleas

Rabbits can be hosts for fleas. It is most important to stress the importance of mxyomatosis vaccination as fleas are the main vector of the virus. Outdoor rabbits that may have contact with wild rabbits may acquire *Spilopsyllus cuniculi* (the rabbit flea) and *Echidnophagis mymecobil* (the stickfast flea). House rabbits may harbour *Ctenocephalides felis felis*, and *Ctenocephalides canis* (the cat and dog fleas).

Treatment: Sprays containing pyrethrin can be used. For house rabbits a spot-on preparation containing 10% imidacloprid (Advantage, Bayer plc) can be used. Program (Novartis Animal Health UK Ltd.) contains lufe-nuron, an insect development inhibitor which prevents flea eggs from developing, and can be given to rabbits. In homes where this method of flea control is used on the cat and dog, this treatment may need to be extended to the house rabbit. The house or hutch can be sprayed with Vet-Kem Acclaim Plus (Sanfoni Animal Health Ltd.) which is an environmental flea spray containing 0.09% w/w S-methoprene and 0.58% permethrin, which kills all stages of the flea life cycle.

Cheyletiella

Cheyletiellosis caused by the non-burrowing mite *Cheyletiella parasitovorax* is the commonest skin condition seen in rabbits. It appears most frequently in the milder warm weather of spring. It is thought to be a common commensal ectoparasite which may cause no problems in normal healthy rabbits, and in many cases infection is asymptomatic. Cheyletiellosis is a zoonotic disease, producing a transient pruritic rash in infected people. It can also be spread to cats and dogs, and this may become more significant as the numbers of house rabbits increase.

Clinical signs: Mild to severe seborrhoeic lesions, usually on the neck or dorsum. The lesions may spread ventrally. The condition is pruritic.

Diagnosis: The mites and skin debris can be picked up on adhesive cellulose tape, and examined under the microscope. The mites are relatively large, and have hooklike accessory mouthparts.

Treatment: The life cycle of *Cheyletiella parasitovorax* is 5 weeks. Ivermectin can be given by subcutaneous injection at a dose of 300–400 µg/kg. Injections can be repeated every 2 weeks, for three doses. Ivermectin is also effective if used topically.

The rabbit can be washed in 1% selenium sulphide (Seleen, Sanfoni Animal Health Ltd.). This shampoo has an antiparasitic action, as well as being beneficial for seborrhoea. The rabbit should be dried with a hair-dryer, and not towelled.

Alternatively the rabbit can be dipped in 0.01% amitraz (Aludex, Hoechst UK Ltd.). The Aludex must be diluted 1:500 to achieve this concentration. Dipping should be repeated weekly for up to 6 weeks.

The hutch should also be well cleaned, and can be sprayed with an environmental flea product such as Vet-Kem Acclaim Plus (Sanfoni Animal Health Ltd.) which contains 0.09% w/w S-methoprene and 0.58% permethrin.

Demodecosis

Infection caused by the mite *Demodex cuniculi* is rare, although it may be seen in immunosuppressed rabbits. The mite is probably present in very low numbers in most rabbits but may only multiply and cause clinical symptoms in the very young or immunosuppressed individuals.

Clinical signs: A moist erythematous dermatitis, with small pustules 2–4 mm in diameter. It is not pruritic.

Diagnosis: Skin scraping. Several skin scrapings may be required to detect the mite. *Demodex cuniculi* is a long thin mite similar to the canine mite, when viewed by microscopy.

Treatment: Ivermectin by weekly subcutaneous injection. A dose of 500 µg/kg may be required to effect a cure. Alternatively the rabbit could be bathed weekly in a 0.01% solution of amitraz (Aludex, Hoechst UK Ltd., diluted 1:500 with water).

Ear mites

Infection with *Psoroptes cuniculi*, the ear mite, is mentioned here, as although it commonly affects the ear, it is capable of causing skin lesions as well.

Clinical signs: Early cases may have mildly pruritic ears, and rabbits can carry low grade infections for long periods of time. More advanced cases have thick yellow–grey crusts in the ears, which are very inflamed. The condition is pruritic. Rarely the lesions may spread across the face and limbs. Crusty lesions have also been reported on the ventral abdomen around the vent. In this site it must be differentiated from treponemiasis (rabbit syphilis).

Diagnosis: Microscopy. The mite will be present in large numbers in the lesions. They may be visible to the naked eye as they may reach 0.7 mm in size. Examination under the microscope reveals their oval body shape, pointed mouthparts and three jointed pedicles with funnel shaped suckers.

Treatment: Ivermectin is given by subcutaneous injection at a dose of 400 µg/kg. The injection should be repeated on two more occasions at fortnightly intervals, as the mite takes 21 days to complete its life cycle. If the ears are to be cleaned the rabbit should be sedated, as removal of the crusts is very painful. The ears and skin can be bathed with dilute chlorhexidine, although there is no actual need to do this because once treatment has begun the crusts will dry up and fall out after a few days. A short-acting corticosteroid can be given by injection to limit the inflammation. A few drops of 1% ivermectin can also be put directly into each ear.

In-contact rabbits should also be treated, and the environment must be disinfected and sprayed with an acaricide, as the female mites can live off the host for several weeks making reinfestation possible.

Fur mite

Leporacarus gibbus (formerly *Listrophorus gibbus*) is another mite commonly found in the fur of rabbits. Its role in the development of dermatitis is uncertain, whether it is a commensal or a pathogen. Unlike *Cheyletiella* there are no reports of it as a zoonosis.

Clinical signs: Alopecia, pruritis and a moist dermatitis. The classic seborrhoea associated with *Cheyletiella* is not a feature. Many infestations may be asymptomatic. The eggs attach to the hair shafts, as do the hatched eggs, and empty larval and nymphal cuticles are left on the hair as the mites develop into adults. This debris gives the coat a 'salt and pepper' appearance.

Diagnosis: Microscopy. The adult female is a similar shape to a flea and much of the cuticle is finely striated. The head is sclerotised, giving it a dark appearance. The legs are short with no clasping adaptations; the mites attach to the hair using membraneous flaps arising from the coxae of the first pair of legs. The males have elongated adanal processes with adanal suckers.

Treatment: Ivermectin injections given weekly for 3 weeks at a dose of 400 µg/kg are effective.

Alternatively, the rabbit can be shampooed in a 0.5% carbaryl shampoo weekly for 4 weeks.

Dichlorvos strips can be hung in the shed as an environmental control. Alternatively, the hutches can be sprayed with a household flea product such as Vet-Kem Acclaim Plus (Sanfoni Animal Health Ltd.) which contains 0.09% w/w S-methoprene and 0.58% permethrin.

Burrowing mites

Other mites that are occasionally found on rabbits are *Notoedres cati*, and *Sarcoptes* species. These mites are zoonotic.

Clinical signs: The lesions are spread over the head, especially around the base of the ears. Infestations by both mites are pruritic.

Diagnosis: Microscopy.

Treatment: Two injections of ivermectin at a dose of 400 µg/kg given a week apart are effective. Alternatively the lesions can be painted with 10% benzyl benzoate every 5 days.

Red fowl mite

Rabbits that are housed with chickens or other fowl may be affected by *Dermanyssus gallinae* which causes intense pruritis.

Ticks

Ticks are occasionally found on rabbits that live outdoors. They are removed in a similar fashion to those on cats and dogs, by applying methylated spirit or petroleum jelly to kill the tick, and then removing with a tick picker.

BACTERIAL SKIN DISEASES

Cutaneous abscesses

Abscesses are very common in rabbits; they may occur anywhere on the body where they are the result of any form of skin trauma, and commonly around the head and neck where they may be associated with dental problems. The nature of rabbit pus is very thick and tenacious, and it is often difficult to effect a cure. However, abscesses are generally not painful, and do not cause the rabbit to feel unwell; rabbits are often able to live with an abscess for months or years whilst on long-term antibiosis.

Clinical signs: A large non-painful swelling, which when aspirated reveals thick yellow purulent material. Microbiological culture often reveals *Staphylococcus aureus* or *Pasteurella multocida*. A culture should always be taken from the wall of the abscess as the centre of the purulent material is likely to be sterile.

Infrequent complications are septicaemia, septic embolus and haematogenous spread.

Treatment: Isolated, well circumscribed abscesses are best treated by complete surgical excision, followed by antibiosis for 2 weeks post surgery. Despite surgery, some abscesses may recur. However, some abscesses are not amenable to surgery. These can be lanced and flushed with a 1%

chlorhexidine solution, povidone-iodine, or an antibiotic solution. The abscess cavity can be packed with an amorphous hydrogel dressing containing glycol and a modified CHC polymer (Intrasite, Smith and Nephew) which will encourage the dissolution of necrotic tissue and promote healing; alternatively it can be packed with calcium hydroxide. Long-term antibiosis is required if the abscess is unable to be completely removed. The most suitable antibiotics are oxytetracycline (Engemycin 5%, Intervet UK Ltd.) given at a dose of 30 mg/kg every 3 days, or enrofloxacin (Baytril, Bayer plc) given in the drinking water at a dilution of 100 mg/litre, or orally at a dose of 10 mg/kg daily. If a rabbit is on long term antibiosis it should be on a healthy diet based on hay and plant fibre, and a probiotic.

In some instances with abscesses of the head area a clindamycin capsule (Antirobe 25 mg, Upjohn Ltd.) can be pricked with a needle and sutured into the abscess cavity to provide a slow-release antibiotic. The rabbit should be simultaneously maintained on a probiotic.

Cephalosporins can be used for short-term therapy if there is a poor response to other antibiotics.

Acute cellulitis

This syndrome is also associated with *Staphylococcus aureus* or *Pasteurella multocida*.

Clinical signs: An inflamed, painful oedematous area, usually around the head or neck. The rabbit is febrile, with a temperature of 40–42.2°C (104–108°F). The lesion may develop into an abscess, or the skin over the area can become necrotic.

Treatment: Aggressive antibiosis. Analgesia should be given to reduce the temperature and manage the pain. Cool baths will also help bring the temperature down.

Blue fur (moist dermatitis)

A moist dermatitis is seen associated with *Pseudomonas aeruginosa*, which affects any skin folds which are kept permanently wet. The skin may be kept wet by saliva or urine, or damp from leaking sipper bottles. The organism is thought to be harboured in drinking bottles, and these should be regularly cleaned.

Clinical signs: The fur classically takes on a blue-green discolouration particularly around the dewlap as the rabbit may 'chin' the water bottle.

Treatment: The area should be bathed and dried. Hair around the lesion should be clipped off. Antibiotics should be used topically, and given parenterally. Enrofloxacin and gentamicin have the best action against *Pseudomonas*. Any dental or urinary problems should be corrected, and cage sanitation improved.

Staphylococcosis

Staphylococcus aureus can cause a pustular dermatitis of young rabbits. Rabbits up to 10 days of age develop moist lesions on the ventral abdomen and medial aspect of the hind legs. Older rabbits (2–4 weeks of age) have numerous small abscesses over the body and a purulent conjunctivitis. Affected rabbits may develop a fatal septicaemia, with abscesses in the liver and other organs. In-contact lactating does may develop a suppurative mastitis, and suckling rabbits may also die as their dams develop agalactia.

Treatment: Antibiotics should be used topically and systemically. As this condition is associated with poor environmental conditions, hutch hygiene should be improved.

Necrobacillosis (Schmorl's disease)

This condition is caused by the bacterium *Fusobacterium necrophorum* and presents as necrotic lesions all over the body, most commonly around the head and lips. The rabbit may also develop multiple abscesses. Affected animals have general malaise and weight loss, and a common sequel is the development of pneumonia. The prognosis is poor.

Treatment: Antibiosis in the early stages. Surgical removal of the abscesses and necrotic tissue may be possible in some cases.

Rabbit syphilis

This disease is caused by *Treponema cuniculi*. The organism is transmitted by direct contact, via doe and buck during mating, and via the doe to her kits at parturition and during lactation. The rabbit spreads its lesions from its genitals to its face and legs as it grooms itself.

Clinical signs: Crusty lesions are found, primarily on the genitalia, but they also appear on the lips, nose, eyelids and perineum. Occasionally lesions may appear on the face and legs alone, whilst the genitalia remain seemingly unaffected. The lesions are not pruritic and begin as oedema, and then form vesicles which burst and become covered with a crust. The inguinal lymph nodes may be enlarged. Affected rabbits are not clinically ill. Other symptoms of reproductive disorders are infertility, stillbirths, neonatal mortality and metritis.

The period between infection and the development of the sores is at least 8 weeks. Symptomless carriers can exist for months before the disease is triggered by stress.

Diagnosis: The condition must be differentiated from ringworm, and ectopic *Psoroptes cuniculi* infection. Deep skin scrapings will determine the bacterium. Silver staining of biopsies will also demonstrate the organism. Serology tests are also available to determine the presence of antibodies.

Treatment: The disease may be self-limiting, but recovered rabbits become symptomless carriers. For treatment procaine penicillin can be used at a dose of 40 000 iu/kg given by intramuscular injection once daily for 7 days. Alternatively an injection can be given once a week for 3 weeks at a dose of 80 000 iu/kg.

Although penicillin is considered dangerous for rabbits because of the potential of developing enterotoxaemia, treatment of syphilis is the exception where it should be used. As long as the rabbit is on a good high fibre diet (hay and greens) with a probiotic, the effects of the antibiotic should be minimal.

All affected, and in-contact rabbits should be treated at the same time.

VIRAL SKIN CONDITIONS

Myxomatosis

This is caused by the myxoma virus which is a pox virus.

Clinical signs

Acute form: The rabbit develops oedematous swellings around the eyes, base of the ears and genitals. The swelling of the genitals is pathognomic for myxomatosis. There is a purulent blepharo-conjunctivitis which progresses to blindness. The rabbit may maintain its appetite initially, but will become anorexic as the disease progresses. Secondary *Pasteurella* pneumonia is very common and the usual cause of death.

Chronic (nodular) form: The rabbit develops oedematous swellings (pseudo-tumours), especially on the ears, nose and paws, 10–15 days after infection. These will spontaneously resolve, although the resultant scabs take longer to disappear.

For further information see Chapter 5.

Warts

Wart-like lesions are caused by the Shope papillomavirus. The warts are usually found on the eyelids and ears. The virus is transmitted from wild rabbits by arthropod vectors. Although these warts are generally benign they may be the precursors to carcinomas.

MISCELLANEOUS SKIN CONDITIONS

Moulting

Rabbits may moult every 3 months. The moults usually alternate between light and heavy shedding. It is very common in Angoras and Cashmeres, and some may go completely bald. Hay must be fed at all times to prevent excessive hair ingestion and to ensure swift passage of any hair through the digestive system. Any loose hair should be removed from the cage every day to limit the amount ingested. Some rabbits may act as if they are very depressed during their moult, and they may become anorexic. They should be tempted with fresh food, in particular chicory, comfrey and spinach. A probiotic can also be given, and this may help stimulate the appetite.

If a rabbit appears to be stuck in moult it is useful to feed some groundsel, as this will often help it to complete the moult. A few drops of codliver oil can be added to the dry food twice a week. A tonic containing vitamin B_1 and minerals such as Metatone (Warner Lambert Consumer Healthcare) is a good conditioner and can be added to the drinking water at a dilution of 20 ml/litre.

Alopecia

(1) Hair loss on the chest and abdomen is common in does during pregnancy and pseudopregnancy, as they pluck their hair to build

nests. Some does can make their skin very sore. If pseudopregnancy is a recurrent problem then ovariohysterectomy is curative. Rarely, nest building has been reported in neutered males.

(2) Hair loss may also be due to barbering. Some rabbits may barber themselves, in which case the hair loss is from the body. Rabbits that are being barbered may have hair loss around the head and dewlap.

   In cases where a dominant rabbit is barbering its companions, the rabbits may need to be segregated. Increasing the fibre content of the diet should reduce barbering, as it will reduce boredom, and provide a constant source of material to chew. Similarly, toys can be introduced to reduce boredom. A single rabbit that is self-barbering will benefit from neutering and pairing with a companion.

   Reducing the light intensity and reducing day length will reduce barbering.

(3) Nutritional. Magnesium deficiency will cause hair loss. To correct this deficiency magnesium oxide can be added to the diet at 0.25%.

Atopy

Clinical signs: Alopecia, pruritis, crusting, erythema, self-trauma of the ears, nose, footpads, thighs, medial hocks and abdomen. There may be accompanying conjunctivitis and epiphora, or epiphora may be the only clinical sign.

Treatment: Parental corticosteroids, and steroid eye drops. The anti-histamine diphenhydramine can also be used. Benadryl elixir can be put in the drinking water at a dilution of 1:45.

Autoimmune skin disease

Facial skin lesions similar to pemphigus have been reported. Lesions predominate around the face, nose, lips and chin. A response is seen to corticosteroid treatment. Prednisolone can be given at an initial dose of 2 mg/kg daily; if a response is seen this dose may be reduced.

Fly strike (blowfly myiasis)

Blowflies are attracted to any damp, soiled areas, and will lay their eggs; in warm, damp conditions these will rapidly hatch into larvae (maggots) in 24 hours. A prime site is the perineum, particularly in overweight rabbits which may have a pouch of skin which remains constantly soiled. Similarly at risk are elderly or disabled rabbits that are unable to clean themselves properly. The larvae burrow under the skin, secreting a chemical similar to local anaesthetic as they go, and the rabbit may be unaware of their presence. The affected rabbit will rapidly become quiet and depressed. The damage to the tissues by the larvae causes hair matting and a moist dermatitis.

Treatment: Initial treatment is aimed at removing the larvae. The rabbit should be sedated if necessary. The area can be sprayed with diluted ivermectin: 0.5 ml Ivomec cattle injection (containing 1% w/v ivermectin) (Merck Sharp and Dohme) can be mixed in a 1 litre of water and used as a spray. The maggots are picked off with forceps.

A single injection of ivermectin at a dose of 400 µg/kg is given sub-cutaneously.

The lesions can be bathed with 1% chlorhexidine, or a 10% povidone–iodine solution.

The skin deficits can be treated with Dermisol cream (Pfizer Ltd.).

The rabbit should also be treated for shock. Fluids can be given sub-cutaneously.

Analgesia must be given. Flunixin meglumine (Finadyne, Schering-Plough Animal Health) can be used at a dose of 1.1 mg/kg by intramuscular injection.

Antibiotics are given, either oxytetracycline at a dose of 30 mg/kg by injection every 3 days or enrofloxacin at a dose of 10 mg/kg orally daily.

For severely affected rabbits euthanasia may be the only option.

Prevention: Owners must be made aware of the importance of checking their rabbit's vents daily for signs of soiling, and for the presence of fly larvae. The rabbit's diet should be improved to contain higher fibre (hay and plant fibre) to reduce the incidence of 'sticky bottom syndrome'. Rabbits with a pouch of skin around the perineum may benefit from a perineal skin fold reduction. If the rabbit's vent area needs to be cleaned regularly it is better to use a skin cleaner which will soften the faeces such as Nolvosan Otic (Willows Francis Veterinary) (contains chlorhexidine), rather than get the whole bottom of the rabbit wet. Shaving the area regularly will help keep the area from becoming soiled.

Attention to cage hygiene should be paramount.

Herbal sprays containing citronella, a natural fly repellent, may be of value, or a pyrethrin-based flea spray can be used around the vent. Other measures to reduce flies in the rabbit's environment should be taken; the use of dichlorvos strips in the shed, or the spraying of the hutches with a household flea spray such as Vet-Kem Acclaim Plus (Sanfoni Animal Health) which contains 0.09% w/w S-methoprene and 0.58% permethrin.

Cuterebra (rabbit warble fly)

In some countries the rabbit warble fly *Cuterebra* will cause a remarkable form of myiasis.

A single larva can pupate in the subcutaneous tissue of a rabbit, and become encapsulated in a large fistulous lesion.

Clinical signs: A swollen mass up to 3 cm in diameter, often around the neck or rump. The swelling will have a single air hole, and the larva can be seen moving inside.

Treatment: Surgical removal of the larva through the air hole. Antibiotics should be given to prevent secondary infection.

Pododermatitis (sore hocks)

Clinical signs: Hair loss, scaling, erythema and ulceration of the skin on the plantar aspect of the metatarsus. Very occasionally the front feet may be affected too. The development of this condition is associated with abrasive or soiled cage floors, in conjunction with obesity and in rabbits that stamp frequently. In house rabbits it may be associated with 'carpet-burn'. It is common in rabbits that only have a thin covering of fur on the foot pad, especially Rex rabbits. The lesions become secondarily infected with *Pasteurella multocida* or *Staphylococcus aureus*, and may develop caseous abscesses. Occasionally the condition may progress to cause osteomyelitis and septicaemia.

Treatment: The lesions should be cleaned with an antiseptic such as povidone–iodine or Clenderm (Univet Ltd.) which contains propylene glycol, organic acids and salicylic acid. Dermisol (Pfizer Ltd.) or Clenderm cream can be applied topically several times a day. If the rabbit will tolerate dressings, the feet may be dressed. Dressings should be changed every 5 days, and once the hock is healing the area can be protected with a lighter covering such as a small sock. A soft, clean surface, either deep dry bedding or towels, should be provided.

The injection of a long-acting steroid under the lesion may be of benefit. The lesions can take weeks to heal.

A tendency towards sore hocks may be inherited, and affected animals should not be bred from.

Skin trauma associated with rabbit rings

Breeders use rings on the hind leg of rabbits for identification purposes. These rings are slipped up the leg and over the hock when the rabbit is young, and as the rabbit matures the ring is unable to slip off. When show rabbits are kept as pets they may put on weight and the leg band can become tight. If unnoticed the band can cut through the skin which exposes the soft tissue structures underneath. In advanced cases there may be swelling of the distal limb.

Treatment: The ring should be removed, and there are special clippers available to enable this to be done in the least traumatic way possible. If the ring is deeply embedded the rabbit may need to be sedated first. The area of damaged tissue should be cleaned with an antiseptic, and a cream such as Dermisol (Pfizer Ltd.) can be applied regularly. Care must be taken to avoid 'fly strike' whilst the tissues are healing.

It is recommended that any rabbit that is not shown should have its ring removed.

Skin tearing

A connective tissue defect similar to the Ehlers–Danlos syndrome has been reported in rabbits.

Perineal skin fold dermatitis

This condition occurs mostly in older does. The excess skin in the perineal region causes a flap which becomes soiled with faeces (caecotrophs) and urine, leading to the development of a moist dermatitis. This soiling leads to an increased risk of 'fly strike'. Some does will develop anorexia and pyrexia.

Treatment: The area can be gently bathed and cleaned daily with a dilute solution of chlorhexidine (Hibiscrub, ICI, UK). The dermatitis can be treated with an antibiotic–corticosteroid cream. The skin can be protected with petroleum jelly, zinc and castor oil cream or talcum powder. Severe cases may benefit from surgery to resect the skin folds.

Procedure for perineal fold reduction: Before surgery it is important to correct the diet to prevent excess caecotroph production and reduce obesity. Any skin infection at the site of surgery must be treated before performing the surgery.

The rabbit is placed in dorsal recumbency, and the skin of the ventral abdomen is clipped and prepared for surgery. A crescent of skin is removed cranial to the genital area, and some of the subcutaneous fat can also be removed. The amount of skin resected should be just enough so that once sutured the ventral skin surface is flat, but not under tension. The incision can be sutured in two layers, an absorbable layer of sutures in the subcutaneous fat to take the tension, and simple interrupted sutures in the skin layer.

Neoplasia

Skin neoplasms include lipomas, squamous cell carcinomas, trichoepitheliomas and basal cell tumours. All of these are slow to metastasise, and surgical excision is curative.

5 THE REPRODUCTIVE SYSTEM

REPRODUCTIVE PARAMETERS

Sexual maturity: 16–24 weeks
Oestrous cycle: induced ovulators
Gestation period: 30–33 days
Litter size: 4–12
Weaning age: 7–8 weeks

SEXUAL MATURITY

Behaviour changes may precede the onset of sexual maturity. A doe may become aggressive, particularly if she lives with another rabbit. She may mount or fight with another rabbit, or start circling and spraying like a buck. She may begin digging or nesting. Small breeds such as the Miniature Lop mature at $3\frac{1}{2}$ months, whereas larger breeds such as the Flemish Giant mature later, between 5 and 7 months. On average, sexual maturity occurs when the rabbit reaches 80% of its adult body weight.

In buck rabbits the testicles generally descend at around 14 weeks of age. After this time they will exhibit mounting behaviour, circling and spraying. Puberty in the buck occurs between 4 and 5 months of age; however, optimum sperm production and reserves are not achieved until 6–7 months.

SEXING

Rabbits can sexed by gentle pressure on the genital orifice which everts the penis or vulva. The penis is extruded as a cylindrical organ, whilst the extruded vulva has a leaf-like appearance. In the male the testicles descend at around 12–14 weeks of age, although they can be retracted into the abdomen if the rabbit is stressed.

Both sexes have two deep inguinal pouches which lie on either side of the genital orifice. These are filled with ceruminous material from the perineal scent glands which are located in these pouches.

OESTRUS

Rabbits are induced ovulators, and do not have regular oestrus cycles. They may have long periods of oestrus, and if mating does not occur the ovarian follicles regress and new follicles mature. This pattern creates a period of receptivity which lasts 12–14 days, followed by 1–2 days when the doe will refuse to mate. When a doe is receptive her vulva is more swollen and often a pink–purple colour. Mating by a buck will trigger ovulation, as will the activity of mounting other does. Ovulation occurs 10–12 hours post-coitus.

MATING

The doe is territorial, and mating is best accomplished if the doe is placed in the buck's hutch, or if they are introduced on neutral territory. Although a single mating is often sufficient stimulus to cause ovulation, it is better to let the buck and doe mate several times over a 30 minute period before the doe is returned to her own hutch. When the buck mates the doe she lifts her hindquarters for him (lordosis). After mating it is normal for the buck to fall off sideways in a spasm and squeal.

PREGNANCY

Following a successful mating the gestation period is 30–33 days, although variations of 29–35 days have been recorded. The foetuses may be palpated by gentle abdominal palpation between 12 and 14 days. In the last week of pregnancy the doe will pull fur out from her chest and abdomen to make a nest. Milk secretion usually commences after parturition. A doe should not have more than three litters in one year.

COMPLICATIONS OF PREGNANCY

Pregnancy toxaemia (ketosis)

Pregnancy toxaemia is rare in rabbits. When seen, this condition is most common in does carrying their first litter. It occurs during the last week of pregnancy, and is most frequently seen in does that are overweight. It has also been seen in pseudopregnant and post-partum rabbits. If the doe becomes anorexic, body fats are broken down to provide energy and the subsequent ketone bodies enter the bloodstream. Fatty liver (hepatic lipidosis) develops. If the doe aborts or gives birth in the early stages the condition may resolve, but if the condition progresses the prognosis is guarded.

Clinical signs: Lethargy, dullness of the eyes, salivation, respiratory distress, convulsions and collapse. The breath may have the classic acetone smell of ketosis. The urine becomes acidic (pH 5–6).

Treatment: Glucose should be given orally, or as a subcutaneous or intraperitoneal injection of 5% glucose. A short-acting corticosteroid injection may be beneficial. The rabbit can be force-fed baby cereal and fruit purée.

Prevention: Young does should not become overfat before breeding. Body fat mass can be reduced by decreasing the concentrate feed, and introducing more roughage in the form of hay and straw. Exercise is important. In a small hutch even placing the food and water sources at opposite ends of the hutch will increase exercise. Any stress which might trigger anorexia in late pregnancy must be avoided.

An electrolyte solution (Lectade, Pfizer Ltd.) or probiotic (Avipro, Vetark Health) containing glucose can be put in the drinking water during the last week of pregnancy for susceptible does.

Pseudopregnancy

Pseudopregnancy may occur after an unsuccessful mating, or following ovulation triggered by the mounting of another doe. This condition usually lasts for about 18 days, and is accompanied by fur plucking, nest building and mammary gland development. The doe may also become aggressive and territorial. If milk is produced, care must be taken that she does not develop mastitis. During this time the doe is unresponsive to being remated. Some does that live alone may be able to self-induce ovulation and can exhibit recurrent false pregnancies; for these ovariohysterectomy is curative, or for the short term a hormone injection can be given. Delvosterone (Intervet UK Ltd.) containing 100 mg/ml proligestone can be given at a dose of 30 mg/kg.

Hydrometra is a rare condition which is thought to arise from a pseudopregnancy which does not reverse, and under the continued influence of progesterone the endometrial glands continue to secrete fluid which accumulates in the uterus (see page 50).

Miscarriage and abortion

Foetal death in the first 3 weeks of gestation will result in resorption, in the last week abortion occurs. There are many possible causes.

(1) *Nutrition*. Obese does may be prone to resorption, or the development of ketosis and subsequent abortion.
    Poor nutrition and low energy intake of the doe is associated with foetal resorption, small litter size and the delivery of weak or dead kits. Deficiencies of vitamin A, E or protein deficiency will result in the loss of litters.
(2) *Infections*. Stillbirths and neonatal mortality can be associated with syphilis (*Treponema cuniculi*). Late term abortion can be caused by *Listeria* infection. *Pasteurella multocida* can cause epididymitis and orchitis in the male, and metritis in the female, and hence reduced fertility of both sexes.
(3) *Other causes*. Stress or trauma. Some rabbits may have a genetic predisposition towards litter loss.

PARTURITION

Parturition generally takes place early in the morning. A normal birth takes around 30 minutes, and the doe eats all the afterbirths and any dead kits. Occasionally the doe may give birth outside the nest. Because it is not a normal response to carry the young into the nest, these young are susceptible to chilling, and must be gently placed in the nest. Uncommonly, some births may span 1–2 days and still result in the birth of normal kits.

PROBLEMS OF PARTURITION

Cannibalism

Cannibalism of the young may occur. This may be accidental, inexperience (first time does), or in response to environmental pressures such as over-crowding. Cannibalism may occur by other does, reverting to their natural survival instincts to cannibalise kits that do not belong to them, to ensure survival of their own line.

Dystocia

Dystocia is uncommon, and generally associated with foetal oversize or malpresentation. Obesity or malnutrition may also predispose to dystocia.

Oxytocin can be given if parturition is delayed, at a dose of 1–2 iu /kg by intramuscular injection. Calcium gluconate can be given orally at a dose of 5–10 ml of a 10% solution if uterine inertia is suspected.

Caesarian section or ovariohysterectomy can be performed on valuable animals.

Uterine prolapse

This is an uncommon condition, but has been recorded associated with dystocia. The prolapsed uterus rapidly becomes engorged with blood, and contaminated with foreign material. Ovariohysterectomy, after first pulling the uterus back into the abdomen, is curative.

CARE OF THE YOUNG

The rabbit is very unusual in the way it cares for its young. Although the young are born naked, blind, helpless and totally dependent on their mother, she visits the nest only once a day, and usually only then for a few minutes. This is an adaptation from the behaviour of wild rabbits that protect their young from predators by concealing the presence of the nest. After each visit the doe will block up the entrance to the nest, and spend her time away from it. The presence of the doe away from the nest does not mean that she has abandoned her young. She is able to do this because her milk is extremely rich and one feed can sustain the young for 24 hours.

Once fed, the young urinate at the top of the nest (they are capable of this from birth and do not require the stimulus of a doe licking them) and then snuggle deep down in the nest until the next feed. 22 hours later they may wake and become active at the top of the nest so that they are ready for the doe's next visit.

DEVELOPMENT OF THE YOUNG

- Day 7: fur begins to grow
- Day 10: eyes open
- Day 12: ears open
- Day 18: leave the nest and begin to eat solid food
- Day 60: fully weaned and independent
- Day 150: sexual maturity

CONDITIONS OF THE UTERUS

Endometrial hyperplasia

The endometrium undergoes changes as the rabbit ages, and the endometrial glands become cystic and hyperplastic. The mammary glands may also become cystic.

Clinical signs: Intermittent haematuria, with the blood being passed at the end of urination. Blood clots may appear with the urine. The rabbit becomes lethargic. The thickened womb may be evident on abdominal palpation, or by radiography. In a breeding doe the first signs may be reduced fertility.

Treatment: Ovariohysterectomy. If necessary histopathology can be performed to differentiate between hyperplasia and adenocarcinoma. Cystic ovaries are commonly associated with this condition.

Uterine adenocarcinoma

This is the most common condition seen in unneutered does. It may occur in rabbits from 2 years of age, and 60–80% of does may be affected by the age of 6 years. It is the principal reason why does should be neutered before 2 years of age. It is thought that falling oestrogen levels in the older doe may be responsible for the development of neoplasia.

Clinical signs: The early stages of the disease are asymptomatic, and many uterine growths are first found during routine hysterectomy in the older doe. As the disease progresses, intermittent haematuria is a feature. The blood associated with uterine pathology generally occurs at the end of urination, rather than mixed evenly with the urine as with diseases of the urinary tract. The presence of blood clots also suggests uterine pathology.

The doe may also become more aggressive, or develop anorexia. The growth is often palpable on abdominal examination, or can be confirmed by radiography. The mammary glands may also become cystic. Metastases are uncommon, but there may be spread to the skin, lungs or liver.

In a breeding doe the first signs may be those of reduced fertility, and foetal loss or resorption.

Treatment: Ovariohysterectomy. As with routine neutering, the uterus should be ligated caudal to the double cervices to ensure the removal of all uterine tissue. A chest radiograph should be taken before surgery to detect metastasis, particularly if the doe is suspected to have an advanced stage of the disease.

The prognosis for does with no signs of metastasis is good following ovariohysterectomy.

Endometrial venous aneurysm

This condition may mimic the clinical signs of uterine adenocarcinoma. The aetiology of this condition is unknown; some does develop large blood-filled uterine horns.

Clinical signs: These are similar to urinary tract infection; the doe may pass blood during or after urination. In the later stages large quantities of blood may be passed. The enlarged womb may be evident on abdominal palpation, or diagnosed by radiography.

Treatment: Ovariohysterectomy.

Hydrometra

This is an uncommon condition, associated with the accumulation of watery fluid within the womb. The aetiology of this condition is unclear, but it is thought to be associated with self-ovulation and pseudopregnancy in the doe. The increase in progesterone stimulates secretory activity of the endometrial cells, and closure of the cervix. If these changes are not reversed at the end of pseudopregnancy, hydrometra can develop.

Clinical signs: Cases may not be presented until the condition is advanced. The uterus may swell until it occupies 80% of the abdominal cavity; hence the rabbit may look normal or obese, whilst actually losing body condition. Eventually the doe becomes anorexic, as the womb presses on the digestive system. Diagnosis is by abdominal palpation and radiography.

Treatment: Ovariohysterectomy.

Endometritis and pyometra

This condition can occur both in pet (unbred) rabbits and breeding does. In the latter it can occur following a recent mating, or following parturition or a pseudopregnancy. Unneutered does housed with castrated bucks that occasionally mount them may have an increased incidence of pyometra. Mild cases of endometritis may show no clinical signs, and still be able to breed.

Pasteurella multocida and *Staphylococcus aureus* are most commonly isolated from cases of pyometra.

Clinical Signs: Cases of pyometra develop anorexia, depression and a creamy vaginal discharge. Haematology may reveal a raised white cell count with a neutrophilia. On abdominal palpation the uterus may feel 'doughy', and will be enlarged on radiography.

Treatment: Ovariohysterectomy, which may be complicated by the presence of adhesions to other organs. If there is a concurrent peritonitis the prognosis is very poor. Fluid therapy is important, and antibiotic therapy should be commenced, preferably based on the results of a bacterial culture and sensitivity.

CONDITIONS OF THE MAMMARY GLANDS

Does have four or five pairs of mammary glands. These glands are absent in the male rabbit.

Mastitis

Mastitis may occur in lactating does that are kept in unsanitary conditions. Teat trauma, injury to the teats, or biting of the nipples will also predispose to the development of mastitis. Mastitis can also occur in association with pseudopregnancy. The causal bacteria are usually *Pasteurella*, *Staphylococcus* and *Streptococcus* spp.

Clinical signs: One or more of the mammary glands will be hot and painful. The affected doe may be pyrexic, anorexic and reject her young. The condition may be fatal for both the doe and her young. Death of the doe is associated with septicaemia.

Treatment: Antibiosis, preferably based on the results of bacterial culture and sensitivity of the milk from affected glands.

The best antibiotics are generally enrofloxacin or a trimethoprim–sulpha combination. Analgesia is most important, and the glands can have warm compresses applied several times daily. The kits should be removed and the doe should be placed in a warm, clean environment. The kits should be hand-reared and not fostered, as fostering may spread the infection to the healthy foster mother.

Cystic mastitis

This is a condition of older does, over the age of 3 years. It occurs in non-breeding does.

It may be associated with uterine hyperplasia or uterine adenocarcinoma.

Clinical signs: One or more glands may be affected. The gland is swollen and bluish in colour. The gland may have a brown serosanguinous discharge from the nipple. The swelling is non-painful. The doe may show other symptoms generally associated with pseudopregnancy such as nest-building and aggression.

Treatment: Ovariohysterectomy. The affected gland can be removed at the same time, although this may not be necessary as the cysts may regress 3–4 weeks after surgery.

Neoplasia

Both mammary papillomas and adenocarcinomas have been recorded. The latter may be present in association with uterine adenocarcinoma. Radiographs should be taken to identify any pulmonary metastases before considering surgery. If the doe is entire, ovariohysterectomy should be advised at the same time.

CONDITIONS OF THE TESTICLES

In male rabbits the testicles descend at around 14 weeks of age. However, as the inguinal canals remain open, the rabbit is able to retract its testicles in times of stress. Cryptorchid males have been recorded.

Epididymitis and orchitis

Infection with *Pasteurella multocida* can cause inflammation and abscessation of one or both testicles. Treatment with antibiotics is unrewarding, and castration should be considered in non-breeding males.

Traumatic wounds

When two buck rabbits fight, they will often attack each other's testicles. Depending upon the degree of trauma caused, some bucks can be sufficiently damaged to require castration.

It is often thought that it is the dominant buck that inflicts the wounds; however, more commonly the dominant buck mounts the submissive buck backwards, and it is the buck underneath that attacks the uppermost buck in self-defence, rather than in aggression. For this reason it is generally advised that bucks are not kept together.

Neoplasia

These are conditions of older bucks. Both testicular seminomas and testicular interstitial cell carcinomas have been recorded. Metastases are unlikely and castration is curative.

RABBIT SYPHILIS (VENT DISEASE)

This disease is caused by *Treponema cuniculi*. The organism is transmitted by direct contact, via doe and buck during mating, and via the doe to her kits at parturition and during lactation. It then spreads from the genitals to the face of an infected rabbit by autoinfection.

Clinical signs: Crusty lesions, primarily on the genitalia, but these also appear on the lips, nose, ears, eyelids and perineum. The lesions are not pruritic. The lesions begin as oedema, and then form vesicles which burst and become covered with a crust. Affected rabbits are not clinically ill.

Reproductive disorders include male infertility, associated with prepucial inflammation. Does develop infertility, metritis, retained afterbirths, still-births and neonatal mortality. The period between infection and the development of the sores is at least 8 weeks.

Diagnosis: The condition must be differentiated from ringworm, and ectopic *Psoroptes cuniculi* infection. Deep scrapings will determine the bacterium. Silver staining of biopsy material will reveal the organism. Serology tests are also available to determine the presence of antibodies.

Treatment: Procaine penicillin at a dose of 40 000 iu/kg given by intra-muscular injection once daily for 7 days. Although penicillin is considered dangerous for rabbits because of the potential of developing enterotox-aemia, treatment of syphilis is the exception where it should be used. As long as the rabbit is on a good high fibre diet (hay and greens) with a probiotic, the effects of the antibiotic should be minimal. All affected and in-contact rabbits should be treated at the same time.

Alternatively 80 000 iu/kg can be given by injection once a week for 3 weeks.

NEUTERING RABBITS

There are many reasons why we should be offering rabbit neutering to our clients as a routine procedure. With the advent of the anaesthetic iso-flurane, rabbits can be anaesthetised safely.

The rabbit does not usually object to isoflurane induction through a face mask, and breath holding does not seem to be a problem. As 98% of the gas is eliminated through the lungs there are no after-effects of anaes-thesia. The concentration of isoflurane can be reduced if the rabbit is sedated before surgery. For bucks, a sedative such as acepromazine can be used; for does, butorphanol will provide both sedation, and post-operative analgesia.

As more veterinary surgeons become familiar with the surgical proce-dures, neutering should no longer be considered a high-risk operation.

Reasons for neutering

The doe

- By the age of 5 years up to 50% (some studies suggest 95%) of does have a chance of uterine adenocarcinoma.

- Uterine infections (pyometra) are common in does over 1 year of age.
- Spaying removes all the behavioural problems associated with sexual maturity, such as nesting, mounting, aggression and mood swings.
- Neutered rabbits are easier to litter train.
- Neutered does can live in the company of bucks (preferably also neutered).
- Prevents unwanted litters.

The buck

- Castration eliminates the behaviour changes associated with sexual maturity such as mounting, spraying and aggression.
- A neutered buck can live with a doe (preferably neutered).
- Neutered bucks are easier to house-train, and smell less (essential if a house rabbit).
- Prevents unwanted breeding.

When to operate

The ideal timing for surgery is as the rabbit reaches sexual maturity. Bucks can be castrated as soon as the testicles descend (around 3–4 months of age). Does can be spayed at 6 months. Some smaller breeds may mature earlier; miniature does may be capable of breeding at 4 months, and may require neutering at this time.

Pre-operative preparation

Rabbits should not be starved before surgery. They are unable to vomit, and studies show that they return to eating post-operatively faster if they have not been starved. Before anaesthesia the rabbits are sedated.

Bucks can be given acepromazine at a dose of 0.1–0.5 mg/kg (0.2 mg/kg is usually adequate).

Does can be sedated with butorphanol at a dose of 0.1 mg/kg. This provides the does with post-operative pain relief, and is not accompanied by the vasodilation of the uterine vessels that is seen with acepromazine.

Ovariohysterectomy

This is performed in a similar fashion to other small animals. A standard midline incision is made into the abdomen. The uterus is located and identified with its duplex cervix and uterine horns. The uterus and ovaries are usually supported by an amount of adipose tissue. The ovaries must be adequately exposed, as often they are buried deep in the adipose tissue. The ovarian vessels must be clamped, and ligated with absorbable suture. The tissues around the ovary are fairly friable, but the blood vessels tend to coagulate readily.

The uterine body should be ligated with a transfixing suture below the double cervix. Care must be taken not to include the ureters which run close to the uterine body at this point. It is often easier to ligate the uterine vessels (which run in the fat alongside the cervix) separately, rather than including them in the transfixing suture.

The peritoneum and abdominal muscles are closed with a simple interrupted absorbable suture, such as vicryl, or a synthetic monofilament suture. The latter provides greater strength and reduces the risk of post-operative herniation. The skin can be closed with a subcuticular absorbable suture (this prevents chewing) or a non-absorbable continuous gentle apposition suture. The latter is less likely to be chewed by the patient than a simple interrupted suture, although as the skin usually heals rapidly as long as the sutures are in for a few days the incision will heal.

Unusual anatomy

During routine surgery unusual uterine anatomy may be found. The commonest abnormality is the absence of a uterine horn. These rabbits have both ovaries, yet only one cervix and uterine horn. The second horn may be blind-ending or absent.

Castration

Castration of the buck is done with a standard canine approach, a midline incision is made anterior to the scrotum. The testicles are pushed into the incision wound, and castration is via the open method. The inguinal ring must be closed to avoid post-operative herniation of the abdominal contents. The large fat pad associated with the epididymis should not be removed, as its presence will help prevent herniation. It is possible to perform a closed castration, but although this method makes herniation less of a risk, it is not possible to ligate the blood vessels as securely, and for this reason an open method is preferred. The skin can be closed with an absorbable material, using either a subcuticular or simple interrupted suture pattern.

Cryptorchids

Genuine cryptorchid males do exist. These can be differentiated from the male that has withdrawn its testicles by the absence of the scrotal sac. Neutering is performed via an abdominal approach as for cryptorchids of other species.

Post-operative care

After surgery the rabbit is given a single antibiotic injection. Does should be given an analgesic, and butorphanol given before surgery will combine analgesia with pre-operative sedation. Further antibiosis or analgesia is unnecessary. The rabbit should be allowed to recover in a warm environment, and allowed access to food and water. For the first few days the rabbit should be bedded on a soft surface, such as 'Vetbed', towels or linoleum, to prevent abrasive bedding materials interfering with the wound. If indicated, suture removal is done 10 days after the surgery.

Pairing, and loss of negative sexual behaviour

The castrated buck can be paired with a doe after 2 weeks. Residual stored sperm should be gone by this time. The average time for negative sexual activity (spraying, mounting and aggression) to start lessening is 2 weeks. The average time for all such behaviour to have gone is 2 months: it may, however, be up to 4 months in larger breeds.

The spayed doe should not be placed with a buck (neutered or unneutered) for 2 weeks, as during this time he could damage her by mounting her. Negative sexual behaviour in the doe lessens and may go completely in 2 weeks.

A neutered pair that live together will occasionally mount each other during their lifetime together and generally form a close pair-bond.

INFERTILITY

(1) *Obesity*. Overweight does fail to breed. They should be put on a hay only diet and encouraged to exercise. They should then have their concentrate feed re-introduced, and mated while they are on a rising plane of nutrition.

(2) *Poor condition*. Does that are underfed will not breed, or may resorb or abort their young. Their diet should be improved, and the protein

content increased. It is also important to have fresh water readily available, as a lack of drinking water may make does resorb their litters. Vitamin E in the form of wheatgerm oil can be added to the concentrate ration. A multivitamin preparation can be given via the drinking water for a few weeks before mating if necessary to improve the doe's condition.

(3) *Concurrent disease*. Any disease process will reduce fertility in either sex. Specific diseases such as syphilis (caused by *Treponema cuniculi*) will cause male infertility associated with prepucial inflammation, and *Pasteurella* infection can cause endometritis in the doe, and epididymitis and orchitis in the buck, resulting in infertility.

(4) *Age*. Does that have not previously had a litter rarely produce after the age of 2 years. From the age of 3 years does may develop uterine hyperplasia or uterine adenocarcinoma, the first sign of which may be reduced fertility and litter size. Older bucks may also become infertile. Testicular neoplasia is rare, but it can cause infertility in aged bucks.

(5) *Compatibility*. Some does just do not like their intended mate. It may help to house the doe in a cage between two bucks, and their scent may stimulate her reproductive system and increase her receptiveness next time she is mated.

(6) *Day length*. Fertility of both sexes decreases as day length decreases.

(7) *Temperature*. Heat stress will lead to reduced fertility.

6 THE NEONATAL RABBIT

DEVELOPMENT OF THE YOUNG

Day 7: fur begins to grow
Day 10: eyes open
Day 12:ears open
Day 18: leave the nest and begin to eat solid food
Day 60: fully weaned and independent
Day 150: sexual maturity

The young are totally dependent upon their mother's milk for the first 10 days of life. They begin eating solid food at 3 weeks of age. They may eat the maternal caecotrophs by day 15, but do not practice caecotrophy until later, at 20 days of age.

DEATH OF YOUNG RABBITS

Sudden loss of one or more kits can be for a variety of reasons, and investigation requires an in-depth assessment of husbandry, nutrition and environmental factors. It is very important that the nest-box is thoroughly cleaned and disinfected before the doe litters, to reduce any bacterial contamination. The doe and her litter must be observed regularly, to ensure she is eating and drinking, and showing no signs of disease. The nest-box should be inspected daily, and any soiled bedding or dead kits removed immediately. Care must be taken to protect the doe and her litter from environmental factors, such as weather extremes, or the stress of predators.

Infectious causes

Bacterial infections are the major causes of loss of neonates. Causal bacteria are *Pasteurella multocida*, *Escherichia coli*, *Staphylococcus aureus* and *Clostridium perfringens*. *Pasteurella* can cause abortion, stillbirth and high neonatal mortality. It is very important that the environment is clean, with no faecal or urine contamination of the nest-box.

Viruses have also been identified as causes of infant mortality. Adenovirus, rotavirus and parvovirus have all been isolated in commercial rabbitries as causal agents.

Coccidia spp. will cause clinical disease in young rabbits. Coccidial infection will lead to weak, anorexic young rabbits.

The doe

Lactation failure

This will result in neonatal death. The doe may develop agalactia if she has concurrent disease such as mastitis, metritis or pododermatitis. Kits that are not feeding will look hunched and dehydrated.

It is important to remember that a doe may only feed the kits once daily, usually in the early morning, so that the absence of the doe from the nest does not necessarily mean that she has abandoned her kits. The kits should be checked daily: well fed kits will have smooth skin and round abdomens.

Mothering instinct

Some does may have poor mothering instincts. This appears to be linked to the hormone prolactin; does with little prolactin appear to be poorer mothers. In some cases the instinct is not apparent until the kits are 2–4 days old, and these kits may require additional support for their first few days.

Occasionally does may not have the instinct to nest-build. If necessary fur should be gently plucked from her, or saved from other does so that a nest can be built for the kits.

Nutrition of the doe

If the doe is poorly fed she may develop agalactia, and the kits will suffer. Anorexia rapidly leads to the development of ketosis, and lactation failure.

Does that are deficient in vitamin E may show symptoms of abortion, stillbirths and neonatal mortality. Levels of vitamin E in the diet can be increased by adding wheatgerm to the feed.

If the doe is overfed she may produce huge quantities of milk, and the young may overfeed and develop milk enterotoxaemia. Excess milk reaches the kit's caecum and allows for bacterial overgrowth and enterotoxaemia. Most at risk are small litters from heavy milk producers.

Scattering

The doe does not instinctively return her young to the nest, and young that stray can readily develop hypothermia and die. It is important to return any young to the nest as soon as possible.

The environment

Predators

The presence of cats or dogs may cause the doe to scatter or crush her young in fright if she is startled.

Weather

Sudden alterations in temperature and draughts must be avoided, as these are a stress which can predispose to disease in both doe and her young.

HAND-REARING OF ORPHANS

Only true orphans need to be hand-reared. It is important to remember that a doe only feeds her young once or twice a day, usually before dawn, and not to mistakenly think that because she is not seen in the nest that she has abandoned her litter. A doe may only spend 5 minutes in the nest all day. The litter of a healthy doe should not be interfered with: if the young are warm and settled and their skin is smooth and unwrinkled then they are being fed. The doe may take 24 hours after littering to come into milk and feed her young. Only young that have not been fed after 48 hours should be given supplementary feeding.

Hand-rearing can be successful, although the younger the baby the more difficult it is. Young rabbits, especially those less than 7 days of age must be kept at a temperature of 27–30°C (80.6–86°F). They can be put in a small box lined with hay and rabbit fur. If it is not possible to obtain rabbit fur, tissues or soft cotton rags can be used. The airing cupboard makes an ideal environment.

The rabbits can be fed on kitten milk substitute, to which is added a probiotic and multivitamin drops or powder. The milk should be gently warmed before it is fed. The kitten milk substitute should be diluted with previously boiled water to the same recommended proportions as for kittens.

Although a doe would only feed her young once a day, as the milk substitute is not as rich as doe's milk, the orphans should be fed 3–5 times a day. Their weight should be closely monitored, and if they fail to gain weight they should be fed more frequently. An approximate guide to the amount of milk an orphan will consume in a day is given below:

Age in days	Milk consumed (ml/day)
1	2
5	12
10	15
15	22
20	27
25	30
30	20
35	Weaned

The orphans can be fed by syringe, or special nursing bottles with teats designed for kittens. If they are started on syringe feeding they cannot be switched to teat feeding as they lose their nursing reflex after 2 days. Syringe feeding may need to be done more frequently than teat feeding as less is consumed at any one feed. Care must be taken to give the milk slowly to avoid aspiration pneumonia, which is invariably fatal. Aspiration pneumonia is less common in young that are teat fed because the natural sucking motion closes the larynx.

After each feed the orphans can be stimulated to urinate and defaecate, by massaging their lower abdomen with cotton wool soaked in warm water. Once the orphans reach 5–6 days of age this may no longer be necessary. It is likely that the kits will be able to urinate unaided from birth, but it is a sensible precaution to stimulate them to do this after feeding. At 3 weeks of age the young will start to nibble hay, and they should be well established on good hay before small quantities of dry food are introduced.

This should prevent weaning enteritis which occurs if young suddenly eat large quantities of dry food and the subsequent carbohydrate and protein overload unbalances their gut flora. Probiotics should be given in the drinking water over the period of weaning to boost the gut flora at this time.

7 THE URINARY SYSTEM

NORMAL URINE COMPOSITION

pH: 8.2–9 (may be as low as 6 in an anorexic rabbit)
SG: 1.003–1.036 (difficult to assess if crystals present)
Crystals: triple phosphate and calcium carbonate are normal
Protein: negative – trace (albuminuria is common in young rabbits)
Glucose: negative – trace
WBCs: rare
Casts: none
RBCs: rare
Bacteria: none to rare

Red urine

This is a common and normal finding in the rabbit. The rabbit is able to excrete porphyrins into the urine which will colour the urine red. It can be distinguished from true haematuria by a dipstick test which will confirm that there is no blood in the urine. Porphyrin excretion in the urine may increase in times of stress. The urine may also become discoloured if the diet is high in carrots or other sources of carotene, as the pigments are not completely broken down by the kidneys and are excreted in the urine. This may colour the urine orange or brown. Eating acorns will similarly lead to the production of red urine. Dehydration will increase the depth of colour, and may occur if water is not readily available, or if it is presented in a container with which the rabbit is unfamiliar. Illness may also lead to a decreased water intake and subsequent concentration of urine.

URINARY TRACT DISORDERS

Haematuria

Haematuria must be first differentiated from 'red urine' by a dipstick test. The differential diagnoses are cystitis, pyelonephritis, urolithiasis, and in the intact female, reproductive disease such as uterine adenoma, adenocarcinoma or endometrial venous aneurysm. The blood associated with urinary tract disease is usually spread evenly in the urine, whereas the blood from reproductive disorders is often produced at the end of, or independently of urination, and may contain blood clots.

Cystitis

Clinical signs: Haematuria, dysuria and pain on urination. There may be perineal soiling.

Diagnosis: This condition must be differentiated from urolithiasis by radiography. Radiography may also indicate the presence of reproductive disorders in the intact female, which do appear to be more common than cystitis. A urine sample should be collected for urinalysis. This can be done by collection into a litter tray, by manual expression, cystocentesis or via catheterisation. Care must be taken when manually palpating the bladder as the bladder wall can be easily bruised or ruptured.

  E. coli and *Pseudomonas* are most commonly isolated in cases of cystitis.

Treatment: Antibiotics, based on urine culture and sensitivity, may need to be given for up to 4 weeks. Drinking should be encouraged, and the rabbit's fluid intake can be increased by offering plenty of fresh vegetables. Dandelions and cleavers are useful feedstuffs as they have diuretic properties. Vitamin C can be given at a dose of 50–100 mg/kg to help heal the damaged bladder. Cranberry tablets, or unsweetened cranberry juice can be used to prevent re-occurrence as the cranberry prevents bacteria sticking to the bladder wall.

Sludgy urine

Because the urine is naturally alkaline, triple phosphate and calcium carbonate crystals readily precipitate out, giving rabbit urine a cloudy appearance. However, if the urine becomes too full of sediment this may lead to urine that is so full of crystals that it is of toothpaste consistency, or ultimately lead to urolithiasis (bladder and kidney stones).

Diets that are high in protein and calcium predispose to crystal development. The rabbit has an unusual calcium metabolism. It appears to have a higher plasma calcium level than other species, and there seems to be a more direct link between dietary calcium and plasma calcium. The plasma levels are controlled by increased excretion in the urine, rather than other homeostatic mechanisms.

Unfortunately urinary acidifiers (used in other species to lower the pH of the urine and aid crystal dissolution) cannot be used in rabbits as they harm the digestive system by altering the intestinal flora. The exception to this is ascorbic acid (vitamin C) which can be added to the drinking water at a dilution of 200 mg/litre.

Clinical signs: Polyuria, dysuria, perineal soiling. Also anorexia and depression. Urinalysis may reveal *E. coli* or *Pseudomonas* infection, and this should be treated with an appropriate antibiotic.

This condition can be corrected by altering the diet to a low protein and low calcium diet. Rabbits with kidney dysfunction also require phosphate restriction.

Obese rabbits should be encouraged to exercise.

Treatment: Some cases may respond to dietary alterations. Antibiosis may be indicated to control secondary infection. Anorexic rabbits will require fluid therapy and analgesia. It is possible to catheterise bucks under sedation in order to flush the 'sludge' from the bladder. If catheterisation is not possible a cystotomy may be necessary to flush the bladder.

Dietary control for calculi prevention

This diet is appropriate for the correction of 'sludgy bladder', and also the long-term management of cases after bladder stone removal. The aim is to produce a diet low in protein and calcium and high in fibre.

(1)   There should be unlimited access to good quality grass hay at all times, as the major fibre provider. Only grass hay should be used; alfalfa hay or blocks must not be given as they are high in calcium.
(2)   Dry or pelleted food (which is high in protein and carbohydrate) should be restricted. The rabbit mix should not contain alfalfa.
(3)   Processed 'treats' (full of carbohydrate and sugar) should be cut out and replaced with fruit treats.

(4) Vegetables and fruit can be slowly introduced from the following list, one at a time. If any item upsets the rabbit it will show diarrhoea 24–48 hours after its introduction, and that fruit or vegetable should be removed from the diet. Once the new regime is fully introduced the rabbit should receive at least half a cup of vegetables per kilogram of body weight daily.

(5) Astringent plants such as blackberry or raspberry leaves can be introduced immediately: they are a good source of fibre and will not cause diarrhoea.

(6) Any vitamin and mineral supplementation should be stopped.

Vegetables: These can be divided into good, moderate and poor sources of calcium. Rabbits receiving some dry mix should be fed almost exclusively on moderate or poor sources only (lists 2 and 3). The calcium in vegetables is in the form of calcium oxalate and is only 49% digestible, compared with the calcium in rabbit pellets which is in the form of calcium carbonate, and up to 80% digestible.

Rabbits on no dry mix can have some vegetables from list 1.

If renal dysfunction or kidney stones are associated problems vegetables with an asterisk should be avoided due to their high phosphorus content.

(1) *Good calcium sources*
     Broccoli leaves
     Chinese cabbage
     Watercress
     Kale
     Dandelions
     Parsley
     Spinach

(2) *Moderate calcium sources*
     Cabbage
     Strawberries
     Radish and radish tops

(3) *Poor calcium sources*
     Carrots*
     Cauliflower
     Cucumber
     Lettuce
     Tomato*

Bananas*
Brussels sprouts
Apples
Pears

Drinking should be encouraged at all times. If necessary a small amount of sweet tasting fruit juice can be added to the drinking water to increase the rabbit's water uptake.

Urolithiasis

Clinical signs: The rabbit may strain to urinate, have genuine haematuria (not 'red urine'), and be stained or wet around the genitals. Pain may be exhibited as teeth grinding, an increased respiration rate and a hunched posture. The rabbit may also be anorexic and lethargic. Litter trained rabbits may lose their litter habits.

Diagnosis: The stone, or stones may be palpable on examination. Radiographs will show the stone and its position; as the uroliths contain primarily calcium they are radiodense. Uroliths are generally calcium oxalate, calcium carbonate, or less frequently ammonium phosphate. Some rabbits may have small stones in the kidneys, and sometimes stones will leave the bladder and become stuck in the urethra. Radiologically the stone will appear as a discrete radiodense mass, in comparison to 'sludgy bladder' when the whole bladder may be filled with radiodense material. Hydronephrosis or hydroureter may occur secondarily, and blood biochemistry may reveal a raised blood urea level.

Treatment: Bladder stones need to be removed surgically, as do stones lodged in the urethra. Stones lodged in the urethra should be retropulsed into the bladder for removal from there. A midline incision is made over the caudal abdomen. The bladder is reflected through the incision and the cystotomy is performed through the dorsal surface of the bladder away from any blood vessels. The bladder should be closed in two layers of simple interrupted sutures with an absorbable suture material such as vicryl.

Post-operative analgesia should be given, and continued for 24–72 hours, until the rabbit is urinating normally. Fluids should be given pre- and post-operatively. Antibiosis is needed, preferably based on the results of a urine culture, and may be required for several weeks.

Prevention: The diet needs to be gradually altered to one of lower calcium content. Fluid intake should be increased, if necessary by adding some sweetened fruit juice to the drinking water, this will help the rabbit diurese itself and keep the urine dilute. Chewable cranberry tablets or cranberry tablets with vitamin C can also be given. The cranberry contains natural ingredients which prevent bacteria adhering to the bladder wall, and the vitamin C helps repair the damaged bladder. These are used in preference to cranberry juice which is often too high in sugar content. The rabbit should be encouraged to exercise, and put on a restricted energy (hay and greens) diet if it is obese. Wild plants such cleavers have a natural diuretic action, and yarrow is of benefit as a urinary antiseptic. Dandelions are also diuretic, but should be given in moderation as they are a source of calcium.

Perineal urine scalding

Although this is most commonly associated with urinary tract disorders, it may occur in association with any condition that makes the rabbit reluctant to move. Spinal pain, pododermatitis, paraplegia, obesity and concurrent illness may all make the rabbit urinate where it is sitting and cause urine scalding. Subsequently the perineum becomes damp and sore. The underlying cause should be investigated and treated. The area should be cleaned daily with a gentle antiseptic such as chlorhexidine and water-resistant antiseptic cream such as zinc and castor oil cream, or Dermisol (Pfizer Ltd.) can be applied to the perineum.

Urinary incontinence

Urinary incontinence may occur in female rabbits after ovariohyster-ectomy. This incontinence is responsive to diethystilbestrol at a dose of 0.5 mg given orally 1–2 times weekly. Phenylpropanolamine (Propalin, Vetquinol UK Ltd.) can also be used at a dose of 6.25–12 mg/rabbit twice a day. Side effects may be inappetence or hyperactivity.

An atonic bladder can be treated with bethanechol, as this increases smooth muscle tone. The dose is 2.5–5 mg orally twice a day.

Incontinence may also be associated with lumbosacral vertebral fractures and dislocations, or central nervous system lesions caused by *Encephalitozoon cuniculi*. Often the loss of litter-box training may be the first sign of arthritis or paresis in the older rabbit. The resultant perineal scalding should be bathed daily with a mild chlorhexidine solution, and a topical antiseptic cream applied.

Ectopic ureters are possible, but rare.

Urolithiasis, cystitis and 'sludgy bladder' will also present as incontinence and perineal soiling.

Urinary catheterisation

Catheterisation is useful for obtaining urine samples, for flushing the bladder of 'sludge', or for contrast radiography. Tom cat catheters may damage the urethral wall, and a softer 3–6 Fr (1–2 mm diameter) flexible catheter or feeding tube should be used. Analgesics should be given after catheter removal. If an indwelling catheter is placed, the rabbit should wear an Elizabethan collar to prevent it chewing at the catheter.

Glycosuria

Glucose may be identified in the urine in times of stress, ketosis and hepatic lipidosis. The latter is possible in any rabbit that has not eaten properly for 48 hours. Diabetes is rare in the rabbit.

The urine should be rechecked on a sample taken at home to rule out stress. Cases of ketosis will have an accompanying ketonuria. A blood sample to check liver enzymes will be necessary to investigate hepatic lipidosis.

THE KIDNEY

Both acute and chronic renal failure can occur in rabbits. Normal biochemical values are as follows:

- Blood urea nitrogen (BUN): 17–24 mg/dl (6.06–8.56 mmol/l)
- Creatinine: 0.5–2.5 mg/dl (44–177 mmol/l)
- Calcium: 5.6–12.5 mg/dl (1.39–3.11 mmol/l)
- Phosphorus: 4–6.9 mg/dl
- Potassium: 3.6–6.9 mg/dl

These values are indicators of renal function and will be raised in acute and chronic renal failure. A raised BUN and creatinine are seen when 50–70% of the renal function is lost.

- Total protein: 5.4–7.5 gm/dl (54–75 g/l)
- Albumin: 2.7–4.6 g/dl (27–46 g/l)

Both these values will be lowered in kidney disease.

Proteinuria is one of the earliest indicators of renal damage, and will appear earlier than a raised BUN or creatinine.

Acute renal failure

Clinical signs: Lethargy, depression, anorexia, polyuria, polydipsia and perineal urine scalding.

Diagnosis: Biochemistry. Urinalysis may reveal proteinuria, haematuria and pyuria. The urine should be cultured to determine if the cause is infectious. *Pasteurella multocida* and *Staphylococcus* are often the causal agents of pyelonephritis.

Treatment: Fluids must be given intravenously to promote diuresis, at a rate of 100 ml/kg per day. If an infectious agent is identified the appropriate antibiotics should be given. Enrofloxacin is a useful antibiotic. Trimethoprim–sulpha combinations and aminoglycocides should be avoided as they are potentially nephrotoxic. The prognosis is guarded.

Comment: The ingestion of nephrotoxins can also cause acute renal failure. Plants that are high in oxalates such as beetroot leaves and aged dock leaves should never be fed. House rabbits are in danger of ingesting lead from items they may find indoors.

Chronic renal failure

This may occur associated with hypercalcaemia and renal calcinosis. Interstitial fibrosis and chronic interstitial nephritis can occur in older rabbits, and fatty degeneration of the kidneys may be seen in obese rabbits.

Clinical signs: Lethargy, depression, anorexia, polydipsia, polyuria and perineal urine scalding.
    Anaemia is a common finding.

Diagnosis: Biochemistry will reveal a raised BUN and creatinine. Urinalysis may show a proteinuria. Haematuria and pyuria are less frequent findings. A glucosuria may also occur with moderate to severe tubular damage. Radiography may demonstrate calcium crystals in the kidneys.

Treatment: Supportive treatment to promote diuresis. Where high blood calcium and renal stones are identified, the diet should be changed as for urolithiasis. Anabolic steroids can be given to reduce the uraemia and improve the appetite; B vitamins should also be given. The prognosis is guarded.

Renal neoplasia

Neoplasia may be identified at post-mortem. Tumours include renal adenomas, adenocarcinomas, nephromas and lymphomas. Embryoma nephromas are the third most common neoplasm in the rabbit, and sometimes can be felt by abdominal palpation.

Renal cysts

Subcapsular cysts can develop in the kidney. They are thought to be an inherited condition. They are of no clinical significance, but an enlarged cystic kidney may be evident on abdominal palpation.

Encephalitozoonosis

This is a common disease caused by the protozoan *Encephalitozoon cuniculi*. The protozoa have a predilection for renal and central nervous tissue. The spores multiply in both sites, and are shed through the urine. The presence of the organism does not necessarily cause disease.

Clinical signs: These generally reflect the central nervous system infection, rather than renal infection. Urinary incontinence may occur as a result of the CNS involvement.

Diagnosis: Antibody titres can be measured. However, it is impossible to distinguish between an active infection, a previous infection or an asymptomatic infection. A negative titre does, however, rule it out of the differential diagnosis. At post-mortem the kidneys are pitted and scarred with multiple white spots on their surface.

8 THE RESPIRATORY SYSTEM

RESPIRATORY DISEASE

Respiratory disease is a major cause of morbidity and mortality in rabbits. Respiratory disease in the rabbit is generally bacterial in origin, rather than viral. *Pasteurella* is the most frequently isolated bacteria, but disease may also be associated with *Bordetella bronchiseptica*, *Staphylococcus aureus*, *Moraxella catarrhalis*, *Mycobacterium*, *Pseudomonas aeruginosa* and *Mycoplasma*.

Rabbits are obligate nose breathers, and respiratory distress can occur readily in cases of upper or lower respiratory tract infection. Mouth breathing indicates severe distress and carries a guarded prognosis.

Dyspnoea may be a symptom of lower respiratory infection, but it may also accompany any cause of abdominal pain, in particular urinary calculi or uterine adenocarcinoma. The patient's respiration should be studied before it is handled and stressed. The normal respiratory rate is 30–60 breaths per minute and is accompanied by nose twitching.

RADIOGRAPHY OF THE THORAX

Radiography of the thorax can be useful in the investigation of respiratory disease. There are several unique features of the rabbit's thorax that make radiographic interpretation different to that of the dog or cat.

The heart lies cranially in the chest close to the thoracic inlet. This makes it impossible to visualise the cranial mediastinum, or to determine the presence of cranial thoracic masses. It is important to extend the forelegs as far forward as possible when taking lateral thoracic radiographs, so that the legs do not obscure the cranial thoracic space. The pleural cavity of the rabbit is small compared with other species, and coupled with a rapid respiration it may be difficult to interpret lung patterns.

73

The presence of body fat, either outside or intra-thoracic can reduce the definition of radiographs, and the use of a grid may improve the detail.

Radiography can determine the presence of heart disease. An enlarged heart is an indicator of cardiac disease, and may be associated with cardiomyopathy, or be due to systemic disease resulting in reduced contractility of the heart. The cranial silhouette of the heart may be difficult to visualise due to the position of the heart in the chest.

Radiology can also help distinguish between upper and lower airway disease. Even if it is not possible to determine the pattern of the lung fields clearly, areas of consolidation and an interstitial pattern in the lungs will indicate lower airway disease.

TRIGGER FACTORS IN DISEASE

There are many factors that can predispose to respiratory disease, and these should be taken into account when investigating a sick rabbit. Nutrition is important, as a hay and fresh vegetable diet can protect against the development of disease. The presence of ammonia either due to poor sanitation, or the feeding of high protein diets, will weaken the respiratory mucosa. Sudden changes in environmental temperature or draughts can trigger infection, and outbreaks are most common in spring and autumn when the temperatures are most variable. The actual environmental temperature is not that important, it is sudden fluctuations that must be avoided. Stress of any sort (age, pregnancy, shows, etc.) is another trigger factor.

In house rabbits the presence of air conditioning or central heating can lower the humidity and increase the amount of airborne dust particles. This may weaken the respiratory mucosa and predispose it to disease. The house rabbit may also be exposed to cigarette smoke which can damage the mucosa.

BACTERIAL DISEASES

Pasteurellosis

Pasteurellosis is caused by the bacteria *Pasteurella multocida*. The disease caused depends upon the virulence of the strain involved, and the resistance of the host. The classical clinical signs of rhinitis ('snuffles') are not seen in rabbits under 12 weeks of age due to the presence of maternal antibodies for the first 8 weeks in endemic groups, and due to the fact that the nasal sinuses of the young rabbit are insufficiently developed to allow colonisation of the bacteria.

The simultaneous presence of *Bordetella bronchiseptica* in the sinuses facilitates *Pasteurella* colonisation.

Not all rabbits that carry *Pasteurella* become ill. Some may spontaneously eliminate the infection, whilst others may become chronic carriers. Healthy rabbits housed with infected rabbits may not get the disease if their resistance is good. Pasteurellosis tends to be a disease of intensively housed rabbits, and is less of a problem in house rabbits.

Clinical signs: The classical symptoms are rhinitis, conjunctivitis, sinusitis and dacrocystitis – the complex referred to as 'snuffles'. The affected rabbit has a white discharge from its nose, and the fur on the medial aspect of the forelegs will be matted and sticky where it wipes its nose. Other symptoms are otitis media and otitis interna (causing 'head tilt', nystagmus and ataxia), pleuropneumonia, pericarditis and tooth root abscesses.

Symptoms of lower respiratory tract infection are anorexia, weight loss, depression and fatigue, with dyspnoea on exertion. These symptoms can occur in the absence of any upper respiratory tract infection. The prognosis for dyspnoeic rabbits is poor.

Abscesses can also form in distant sites causing testicular abscesses, endometritis, and pyometra. Septicaemia caused by *Pasteurella* is one of the commonest causes of sudden death, which may occur following stress, with few preceding clinical signs.

Transmission: The most common form of transmission is by direct contact, and by inhalation of airborne droplets containing bacteria. The bacteria can survive for several days in moist secretions and water. Indirect spread can occur via bowls and drinkers contaminated by nasal secretions. Rabbits can only sneeze to a distance of 2 metres (about 6 feet), and infective droplets can be spread over this distance.

The bacteria enter through the nares or through open wounds. The infection then spreads to neighbouring tissues, or to distant sites haematogenously. Infection travels from the nares to the middle ear via the eustachian tube.

Rarely, the bacterium can be transferred at mating, or parturition.

Diagnosis: Nasal swabs of rabbits with 'snuffles' may reveal *Pasteurella*. However, in the case of infection at distant sites nasal culture may be negative. *Pasteurella* can also be cultured from the respiratory tracts of healthy rabbits.

Serology (ELISA) can be done. A high antibody titre may imply a chronic carrier state rather than the elimination of infection, so the results of serology and culture must be assessed alongside the clinical signs.

Radiography may be necessary to determine the extent of respiratory disease. In cases of otitis the tympanic bullae which are normally thin-walled and hollow develop an increased soft tissue opacity and thicker walls.

Post-mortem examination of cases of sudden death associated with *Pasteurella* have petechiation and microscopic abscesses throughout the viscera.

Treatment: It is not usually possible to cure infected rabbits, but it may be possible to stabilise them with antibiotics so that they can live with chronic disease. Antibiotics are frequently needed for long periods, often as long as 6 months to 1 year. A culture should be done where possible.

Pasteurella is generally sensitive to enrofloxacin, chloramphenicol, gentamycin, tetracycline and trimethoprim–sulpha drugs. Enrofloxacin is the drug of choice for long term medication, and can be given initially at a dose of 5–15 mg/kg twice daily, and then given orally at 10 mg/kg daily, or via the drinking water at a concentration of 50–100 mg/litre.

Severe cases can be given procaine penicillin at a dose of 20 000–60 000 iu daily for 5 days by intramuscular injection.

Other drugs that can be used as an adjunct to therapy are analgesics (NSAID), antihistamines (diphenhydramine, e.g. Benadryl, Parke Davis and Co. Ltd.), and mentholated vapour rubs to ease congestion. Eye preparations containing antibiotic can also be used. Gentamicin can be used as ear or nasal drops as indicated.

Fluids are important, and can be given subcutaneously at a rate of 100 ml/kg per day in debilitated rabbits. The fluids will help hydrate the mucus produced by the nasal epithelium and facilitate its excretion.

A good diet is very important, and the addition of vitamin C may improve recovery. The rabbit should be kept at a constant environmental temperature of 16°C (about 60°F), with a relative humidity of between 50 and 70%.

Prevention: Good husbandry is very important. A good diet of hay and fresh greens will protect against infection by improving the rabbit's resistance. In a group where *Pasteurella* is endemic, early weaning at 4–5 weeks will remove the young before they become infected. However, weaning at this time can be stressful. If weaning later, antibiotics can be given over the time of weaning, and tetracycline can be given in the drinking water at a dilution of 250 mg/litre.

Rabbits can sneeze over a distance of 2 metres (about 6 feet), and where possible hutches should be spaced apart to prevent spread by infective droplets.

Vaccination with a sheep vaccine may help control the disease, but will not cure it. Pastacidin (Hoechst Roussel Vet Ltd.) contains killed bacterial cells of *Pasteurella*. A dose of 0.25–0.5 ml (young rabbits) or 0.5–1 ml (adults) can be given by subcutaneous injection, and the treatment repeated after 2–3 weeks. Does can be boosted just before mating so that they will confer maternal immunity to their young for the first 8 weeks of life. Young stock can be given their first injection after weaning. Bucks can be given a booster every 6 months.

Vaccination is good at stimulating a non-specific immunity and may give the rabbit a better resistance against other infections.

Comment: As not all respiratory infections are *Pasteurella*, the nasal discharge must be cultured if there is a history of a previous poor response to antibiotics.

Bordetella bronchiseptica

Many rabbits carry *Bordetella bronchiseptica* in their upper respiratory tract. It is not associated with disease, but its presence may increase the rabbit's susceptibility to *Pasteurella* infection. It can be transmitted to guinea pigs and it is pathogenic in this species; *B. bronchiseptica* infection should be considered if rabbits are housed with guinea pigs.

Staphylococcus aureus

This bacterium is carried in the upper respiratory tract of healthy rabbits, and it is also carried by humans. It may cause disease depending upon the virulence of the strain and host resistance. It is the commonest cause of conjunctivitis, and may also be associated with the development of a nasal discharge and pneumonia. The pneumonia is associated with the formation of multiple small abscesses in the lungs, in comparison with *Pasteurella* pneumonia which causes a purulent pleuropneumonia.

When possible, treatment should be based on a bacterial culture and sensitivity test. If this is not possible the best antibiotics are enrofloxacin or a trimethoprim–sulpha combination. Antibiotics will reduce the clinical signs but may not eliminate the organism.

Eye ointment containing fusidic acid (Fucithalmic, Leo Laboratories Ltd.) is active against *Staphylococcus* and is useful in cases of conjunctivitis.

Moraxella catarrhalis (formerly Neisseria)

This bacterium is commonly carried in the upper respiratory tract of rabbits. It is not considered a primary pathogen, but may cause infection as an opportunist if the respiratory mucosa is already diseased. No treatment is necessary if it is isolated from the nares of a healthy rabbit.

Pseudomonas

Pseudomonas is not a normal inhabitant of the respiratory tract, and if it is isolated it should be considered pathogenic. It is an opportunist bacterium which will colonise weakened respiratory mucosa, and predisposing environmental factors must be investigated.

VIRUSES

Viral causes of respiratory disease are not well documented, and thought not to be a common problem. The myxoma virus causing myxomatosis is accompanied by respiratory symptoms only if there is secondary bacterial infection in chronic cases. Mild cases of haemorrhagic viral disease (HVD) which recover may go on to develop secondary respiratory disease. HVD causes multiple lung haemorrhages, and death in its more acute form.

OTHER CAUSES OF RESPIRATORY DISEASE

Allergies

Rabbits can develop epiphora, rhinitis, sneezing and bronchitis in response to inhaled allergens. In rabbits kept outdoors in hutches these allergens may be pollens, dusty hay or wood shavings. House rabbits are likely to be exposed to many different aerosols such as furniture polish, air fresheners and perfumes, and these should be taken into consideration. House rabbits may also be exposed to cigarette smoke which may predispose them to respiratory disease.

Treatment: If the allergen can be identified, it should be removed from the environment. If this is not possible then the rabbit can be given anti-histamines or corticosteroids to reduce the symptoms. Care should be taken with the administration of corticosteroids over a long period of time as the immunosuppression caused can trigger latent *Pasteurella* infection.

The antihistamine diphenhydramine can be put in the drinking water, e.g. Benadryl elixir (Parke Davis UK Ltd.) at a dilution of 1:45 in the drinking water daily.

Mandibular prognathism

Short nosed breeds, such as the Netherland Dwarf and the Lop breeds, may snuffle, particularly when they are eating. This is associated with the shortening of the nasal passages, as seen in brachycephalic breeds of dog. This snuffling is not accompanied by a nasal discharge, and is not of clinical significance.

Neoplasia

The lungs are a site of metastasis for uterine adenocarcinoma. Clinical signs include weight loss, dyspnoea and lethargy.

Thymomas can also occur. The thymus persists into adult life and occupies the cranial thoracic area, extending forwards into the thoracic inlet. Thymomas may be difficult to diagnose on radiography as the heart is positioned cranially in the chest, and the cranial thoracic area is often poorly defined due to the presence of fat and the superimposed shadow of the forelegs. No treatment is possible.

CARDIAC DISEASE

Heart disease is a relatively rare finding in rabbits. However, as rabbits are kept in better conditions with good medical care their life expectancy is longer than previously. This increases the incidence of heart failure and arteriosclerosis.

Arteriosclerosis is caused by excess vitamin D in the diet, leading to mineralisation of the aortic arch and thoracic aorta. Aortic atherosclerosis is associated with elevated blood cholesterol (normally 10–80 mg/dl). Cholesterol levels are variable, depending upon age, sex, breed and the time of day. There may be an inherited tendency in some breeds of rabbit towards high cholesterol levels.

Cardiomyopathy has been seen in association with coronavirus infection.

Clinical signs: Increased respiratory rate, mouth breathing, wheezy chest sounds, hind leg weakness, anorexia and chronic weight loss. Rabbits in severe respiratory distress will have an arrhythmic heart rate (more than 200 beats per minute) and cyanosed mucous membranes. On radiography there will be pleural effusion and pulmonary oedema. ECGs are not always helpful in the diagnosis of heart disease.

Treatment: Rabbits in acute respiratory distress should be given oxygen, either by face mask, or in an oxygen tent or cage. An intramuscular injection of frusemide can be given at a dose of 4 mg/kg.

Maintenance therapy is symptomatic with diuretics and bronchodilators.

- Frusemide can be given at a dose of 2–5 mg/kg orally twice a day.
- Benazepril hydrochloride (an ACE inhibitor) can be given at a dose of 0.25–0.5 mg/kg daily orally.

SUDDEN DEATH

Rabbits may die suddenly when stressed. This is particularly true of rabbits that are kept in small hutches all their lives with no opportunity to exercise and develop strong heart muscle and cardiovascular fitness. The surge of adrenaline that is produced in stressful situations may be more than the weak heart muscle can cope with. To prevent this occurring all rabbits should be allowed 1–4 hours of free exercise a day to maintain fitness.

House rabbits can die of cardiogenic shock if they chew through electric wires. For this reason all wires should be 'bunny-proofed' or the rabbit should be supervised at all times when it has free run of the house.

9 THE DIGESTIVE SYSTEM

PHYSIOLOGY

The rabbit digestive system is a complex one, and a balanced diet with an emphasis on plant fibre is required to ensure normal gut motility.

The stomach holds all the food, and effectively sterilises it with its pH of 1–2. The food then passes through the small intestine where all the nutrients are absorbed. The ingesta then pass into the large intestine, where the larger pieces of indigestible fibre are processed into hard faecal pellets, whilst all smaller particles are moved backwards (by muscle fibres called haustrae) into the caecum for fermentation.

The caecum ferments the smaller particles (cellulose), and bacteria produce B complex vitamins and volatile fatty acids. This material forms the small, soft pellets called caecotrophs which are coated with mucus and are consumed by the rabbit directly from the anus by the process of coprophagy.

- High fibre diets stimulate the rapid movement of ingesta through the gastrointestinal tract. Low residue diets lead to reduced gut motility, and impaction secondary to gastric stasis is more common. It is the coarse indigestible fibre (lignocellulose) which is most important.
- Diets high in sugar and starch will exceed the small intestine's capacity to absorb them, and sugar and starch in the caecum may lead to a proliferation of micro-organisms which cause enterotoxaemia.
- The pH of the stomach may rise in anorexia or disease.
- A compact food-ball of concentrated dry food may not be effectively sterilised, allowing micro-organisms to pass further down the digestive tract.

Physiological development of the digestive system

In the neonate, the stomach pH is 5–6.5. For the first 21 days of its life the kit is able to produce an antimicrobial fatty acid from its gastric lining (the stomach oil) in response to the doe's milk. Hand-reared rabbits are unable to produce this protective fatty acid. This protection wanes at 21 days, and the pH of the stomach gradually drops to pH 1–2. It is during this transition that bacteria are able to pass through the stomach and colonise the hind-gut, and therefore also the time that the young rabbit is most vulnerable to enteric pathogens. The kit is totally dependent on milk up to 10 days of age. At 15 days of age the kit begins to ingest maternal caecotrophs, and at 20 days of age it begins to practice caecotrophy.

THE MOUTH

Oral papillomatosis

This is a rare condition caused by a papilloma virus. White lesions occur on the underside of the tongue and may become ulcerated. The condition is usually self-limiting and the lesions regress after several weeks.

Oral ulceration

Ulceration in the mouth is common, and the first presenting signs are salivation and anorexia. The ulcerations are caused by the overgrowth of the cheek teeth (see Chapter 11). The lower molars cause lingual ulceration, whilst spurs from the upper molars generally grow laterally and cause buccal ulceration. Treatment is aimed at correcting the underlying dental problem.

THE STOMACH AND SMALL INTESTINE

Gastric stasis

If gastric motility is reduced, ingesta remains in the stomach for longer. If hair is mixed up with the ingesta, a solid impacted mass forms as the stomach contents dehydrate. Such a 'hairball' is not a primary condition, but secondary to reduced gut motility.

Reduced gut motility is usually the result of feeding a low fibre diet. In these cases the stomach and caecum empty very slowly. The rabbit produces less and less pellets, and will stop eating. A mass of impacted ingesta is generally palpable in the stomach and caecum. Radiographic signs include a classic 'halo' of gas around a ball of impacted foodstuff in the stomach.

Treatment

- Fluids can be given by subcutaneous injection, and orally (with an electrolyte solution).
- Pineapple juice will provide fluids, and the enzyme (bromelain) will help break down the mucus that binds the hair and ingesta together in the impaction. Up to 10 ml can be given three times a day.
- A cat laxative (Katalax, C-Vet Veterinary Products) can be given 30 minutes after the pineapple juice. The dose is 3 ml twice daily. Alternatively liquid paraffin or Milpar (Stirling Health, UK Ltd.) can be given at a dose of 5 ml two or three times daily.
- Metoclopramide (Emequell, Pfizer Ltd.) given by subcutaneous injection will stimulate gastric emptying and gastric motility. The treatment can be followed up by giving Emequell tablets twice daily: dose 0.2–1 mg/kg.
- Cisapride (Prepulsid, Janssen, UK) 0.5–1 mg/kg can be given orally every 8–24 hours. This is another motility drug with a different mode of action to Emequell, and both drugs can be given simultaneously.
- Vitamin B injection, as ingestion of caecotrophes is unlikely to be taking place.
- Leafy greens should be offered, especially those of laxative plants, e.g. dandelions. Also offer good quality hay.
- Advanced cases may require surgery to relieve the impaction, but only if symptomatic treatment and supportive care have made no difference. Depending upon the condition of the rabbit it may take 2–3 days for the medical treatment to stimulate gastrointestinal motility, and only when this fails should surgery be considered.
- Analgesia.
- Antibiosis with a trimethoprim–sulpha combination at a dose of 30 mg/ kg twice daily will help prevent bacterial overgrowth.

Prevention: A high fibre diet should be fed of good hay and a reduced pelleted ration. The pellets should contain a minimum of 18% fibre and less than 16% protein. A variety of vegetables should be gradually introduced into the diet, and then included on a daily basis. Starch and fat should be minimised (no legumes, grains, etc.) Rabbits should be allowed to exercise daily.

Hairballs (trichobezoars)

Hairballs are no longer thought to be a primary condition, but rather to occur secondary to gut stasis. There are, however, predisposing factors that make their formation most likely.

- A low fibre diet (high fibre diets stimulate the rapid passage of food through the digestive tract, taking the hair with it).
- Low exercise.
- Long haired breeds, or any breed during an excessive moult. (Rabbits under 7 months of age are unlikely to suffer hairballs as it is only at this time that they develop a full hair coat.)
- Mutual grooming of a companion that is moulting.
- House rabbits can ingest other fibres such as carpet which will cause a similar impaction.

Treatment: See Gastric stasis.

Prevention: A high fibre diet and increased exercise. Exercise stimulates peristalsis (gut motility) and improves the passage of food through the gut. The grooming of long-haired breeds and those in heavy moult will help.

Gastric intestinal obstruction

Obstructions may occur at the pylorus of the stomach, or in the duodenum. The cause of the obstruction may be matted hair (matted before ingestion), plastic foreign bodies, or ingested carpet. Ingestion of clay cat litter can also cause obstruction.

Clinical signs: Sudden onset gastric pain and bloating. On radiography, gas accumulation will be evident cranial to the obstruction.

Treatment: An analgesic must be given such as buprenorphine at a dose of 0.01–0.05 mg/kg by intramuscular injection. A dose of rapid acting corticosteroid is indicated to counteract shock. Fluids should be given, preferably intravenously.

The obstruction must be removed surgically.

Intussusception

This is uncommon, but may occur in young rabbits in association with enteritis, or in older rabbits associated with a foreign body.

Clinical signs: Anorexia, and a cessation of droppings. The intussusception is generally palpable on abdominal examination, and radiographs will demonstrate the build up of gas cranial to it.

Treatment: Surgical correction. Warmed fluids can be given intraperitoneally as the abdomen is being closed.

THE CAECUM

In proportion to its bodyweight the rabbit has the largest caecum of any living mammal. The caecum is the fermenting vat of the digestive system. It ferments small particles of cellulose, and bacteria produce B vitamins and volatile fatty acids. The dominant bacteria in the caecum are Bacteroides with small amounts of *Clostridium* sp., *E. coli* and *Streptococcus faecalis*. Bacteroides are Gram-negative cellulolytic anaerobes. The products of this digestion are soft small pellets called caecotrophs which are redigested by the rabbit. These caecotrophs are encapsulated in a mucilaginous coating to survive the passage through the stomach's acidity and are digested and absorbed in the small intestine.

Normal caecal pH is between 5.9 and 6.8. Normal flora decrease when the caecal pH is out of range (such as acidification when excessive fermentable carbohydrates are fed), then *Clostridia* sp. can proliferate and cause enteritis. The populations of *Clostridia* and *E. coli* rise in direct proportion to a falling fibre content of the diet.

Pinworms (*Passalurus*) are now considered to be normal inhabitants of the caecum. Similarly Saccharomycetaceae yeasts are considered nonpathogenic, and their numbers fall as the fibre content of the diet increases.

Excess caecotrophs ('sticky bottom syndrome')

Some diets, particularly those that are high in protein, low in fibre and high in carbohydrate or sugar, will cause the rabbit to produce more caecal faeces than it needs, and hence develop a 'sticky bottom'. If the rabbit is overfed, particularly if it is on a high protein diet, it may lose the urge to practice coprophagy. Large rabbits kept in small hutches may not have space to stand on their hind legs and reach their anus. Caecal faeces may also build up if the rabbit is unable to perform coprophagy, if for example it is overweight, has an excessive dewlap, has incisor or molar malocclusion (which will make coprophagy uncomfortable) or has arthritis and spinal pain.

Dietary reform means changing the rabbit over to a high fibre, low protein and low carbohydrate diet, which actually provides a more natural diet, and one closer to that of their relatives, the wild rabbit. The rabbit's digestive system works at its best when it has to break down plant fibres.

(1) There should be unlimited access to good quality grass hay at all times, as the major fibre provider.
(2) Dry or pelleted food (which is high in protein and carbohydrate) should be restricted.
(3) Processed 'treats' (full of carbohydrate and sugar) should be cut out and replaced with fruit treats.
(4) Vegetables and fruit can be slowly introduced from the following list, one at a time. If any item upsets the rabbit it will show diarrhoea 24–48 hours after its introduction, and that fruit or vegetable should be removed from the diet. Once the new regime is fully introduced the rabbit should receive at least $\frac{1}{2}$ cup of vegetables per kilogram of body weight daily.

Vegetables: broccoli, brussels sprouts and sprout tops, cabbage and cabbage types, spring greens etc., carrot and carrot tops, celery, clover, dandelions (leaves and flowers) – use sparingly, kale, mint, parsley, radish tops, spinach, watercress.

Fruit: small amounts of apple, peach, pear, melon, pineapple, plums, strawberries and tomatoes can be added or used as 'treats'.
(5) Astringent plants such as blackberry or raspberry leaves can be introduced immediately; they are a good source of fibre and will not cause diarrhoea.

Hay alone should be fed first, provided the rabbit is used to eating hay, otherwise it must learn to eat hay before everything else is withdrawn. After the faeces have been normal for a week, the greens can be introduced slowly. It may take a week, or up to several months on hay only before the faeces are normal.

Caecal impaction/tympany

If the passage of ingesta is slow, and if the diet is a low fibre one, this will result in the build-up of food material in the caecum. Prolonged fermentation of this material will lead to tympany, and if there are excess sugars or starch present this will alter the pH of the caecum and allow a build up of the bacterium *Clostridium spiriformes* which can lead to a fatal enterotoxaemia.

Caecal impaction can be easily palpated per abdomen.

Treatment:

- Gut motility must be encouraged as for gastric stasis, with metoclopramide (Emequell, Pfizer Ltd.) and cisapride (Prepulsid, Janssen UK Ltd.).
- A probiotic such as Avipro (Vetark Health), provides *Lactobacillus*. Although *Lactobacillus* and *Acidophilus* are not significant microorganisms in the rabbit caecum, in situations where a build-up of harmful bacteria is likely, their presence may help overpower the *Clostridium* spp. The *Lactobacillus* is encapsulated, and able to pass through the stomach's acidity into the caecum.

Transfaunation

This describes the process of giving a faecal cocktail from a healthy rabbit to a sick one, in order to replace the natural micro-organisms, supply B vitamins, and stimulate the appetite.

A buster (Elizabethan) collar is put around the healthy rabbit to prevent coprophagy, and some caecal pellets are harvested overnight. One faecal pellet can be mixed with 5 ml warm water, and administered orally by syringe or stomach tube.

Enteritis

Enteritis (diarrhoea) can occur for many reasons; a dietary change, bacterial, protozoal, viral, following antibiotic use, or at times of stress. Specific syndromes are detailed in this section.

Rabbits with diarrhoea often have a higher stomach pH (3–7), enabling bacteria to pass to the hind-gut.

Basic treatment protocol

Whatever the cause of enteritis, the principles of treatment remain the same. Specific treatments are detailed in the following sections.

- *Nursing.* The patient should be kept in warm, clean, stress-free surroundings.
- *Fluid replacement.* Aim to provide between 50 and 100 ml/kg per day in divided doses. Fluids (lactated Ringer's solution (Hartmann's solution)) can be given by intravenous or subcutaneous injection. Oral fluid replacement (Lectade, Pfizer Ltd.) can be given by syringe or stomach tube.

- *Stimulate normal gut motility*. Metoclopramide (Emequell, Pfizer Ltd.) can be given at a dose of 0.5 mg/kg up to four times a day; this stimulates gastric emptying, and should lead to an improvement of caecal motility.
- *Antibiotics*.
- *Analgesia*. Carprophen (Rimadyl, Pfizer Animal Health) at a dose of 1.5–2 mg/kg.
- *Probiotics*. Avipro (Vetark Health) contains *Lactobacillus* which can temporarily colonise the caecum and protect against the multiplication of harmful bacteria.
- *Transfaunation*. The permanent way to repopulate the caecum.
- *Diet*. Astringent plants such as shepherd's purse, blackberry and raspberry leaves can be given. The fibre content of the diet should be increased: leave off dry food and feed good quality hay. Herbal powders made from astringent plants can be used.
- *Kaolin* given as a kaolin or kaolin–pectin mixture orally may help bind up the liquid faeces.

Neonatal (colibacillosis)

- Affects rabbits of 1–14 days of age.

Diarrhoea in neonates is commonly caused by an enteropathogenic *Escherichia coli*. Rabbit strains of *E. coli* do not produce enterotoxins as they do in other species.

Clinical signs: A yellow, watery diarrhoea which stains the perineum and abdomen. The morbidity and mortality within a litter may reach 100%.

Pathology: At post-mortem there is milk in the stomach, whilst the rest of the gastrointestinal tract is filled with watery contents. The finding of *E. coli* is significant in rabbits under 2 weeks of age, as it is not a normal component of the gastrointestinal flora at this age.

Treatment: Early cases may respond to antibiotic therapy (either trimethoprim–sulpha combinations or neomycin) fluids and a probiotic.

Subsequent litters from the same doe may have passive immunity. As poor husbandry and sanitation are predisposing factors for colibacillosis, these must be investigated and improved as necessary.

Weaning enteritis

- Affects rabbits of 4–8 weeks of age.

At weaning the body undergoes various physiological changes. In suckling rabbits the pH of the stomach is between 3 and 6.5, whereas in the adult the pH is 1–2. For the first 21 days of its life the kit is protected by an antimicrobial fatty acid (the stomach oil) which is produced by the gastric lining in the presence of doe's milk and which controls its gastrointestinal microflora. After 21 days this protective factor wanes and the hind gut becomes populated with bacteria. A high stomach pH means that harmful bacteria may be able to pass through the stomach into the caecum and small intestines, and cause enteritis. In association with this, if the weanling consumes large amounts of high energy food, this will provide fuel for the multiplication of harmful bacteria (*Clostridium spiriformes*) in the caecum. At this time the rabbit is more dependent than ever on a healthy population of micro-organisms in the caecum.

Clinical signs: Rabbits of 4–8 weeks of age are commonly affected. There is profuse diarrhoea, dehydration and a rough hair coat. Mortality may be 100%.

Pathology: Lesions are commonly seen in the caecum. There is haemorrhagic inflammation of the caecum which is filled with watery or mucoid blood-tinged fluid.

Treatment: Fluid replacement with subcutaneous fluids (lactated Ringer's solution (Hartmann's solution)); oral fluids with an electrolyte solution, e.g. Lectade (Pfizer Ltd.). Fluid replacement should be maintained at a rate of 50–100 ml/kg per day in divided doses. A probiotic such as Avipro (Vetark Health) can be given to populate the gut with *Lactobacillus* and *Enterococcus*, or the gut can be repopulated with caecal pellets from a healthy rabbit (see Transfaunation).

A broad-spectrum antibiotic can be given, e.g. sulphonamides or Neobiotic aquadrops (Upjohn Ltd.) which contain neomycin.

During an outbreak the pellet ration should be decreased, and unlimited good quality hay offered. Water should be available at all times.

Prevention: During the period of weaning plenty of fibre (hay) should be available. The concentrate ration should be introduced slowly so that there is not a flood of energy and nutrients into the caecum which may destroy the balance of micro-organisms. A probiotic (Avipro, Vetark Health) can be dissolved in the water during this stressful time.

Stress should be minimised. In the case of intensive breeding this may mean the provision of larger hutches, with a separate nest area to avoid overcrowding. It may be advisable to leave the young with the doe longer before weaning, giving their immune system longer to develop. When weaning the doe should be removed from the young, rather than the young being taken away. This avoids the double stress on the young of a new environment and no mother.

Concurrent infection with coccidia should be avoided.

Mucoid enteritis

- Affects rabbits of 7–14 weeks of age.

The exact cause of mucoid enteropathy is unknown, but its aetiology is similar to that of weaning enteritis. It is caused by changes in caecal pH that are associated with disruption of the normal caecal flora. It is a disease of young rabbits, just beyond weaning age (7–14 weeks) which is the age when the caecal microflora are becoming established, and are at their most vulnerable. Mortality is common. In up to 60% of cases there may be an accompanying pneumonia.

In older rabbits an enteritis associated with mucus production is more likely to be part of the 'enteritis complex' rather than classic 'mucoid enteritis' and mortality is lower.

Mucoid enteritis is rarely seen in rabbitries that feed a high fibre diet and avoid excesses of grains, proteins and fats.

Clinical signs: Anorexia, lethargy, weight loss, diarrhoea, polydipsia, caecal impaction and an excessive production of mucus by the caecum.

Treatment: As for weaning enteritis.

- Fluid replacement, either via subcutaneous injection, or orally with an electrolyte solution such as Lectade (Pfizer Ltd.).
- A high fibre diet is offered, good grass hay or alfalfa. Vegetable baby food can be given orally by syringe feeding.
- Metoclopramide (Emequell, Pfizer Ltd.) can be given at a dose of 0.5 mg/kg up to four times a day: this stimulates gastric emptying, and should lead to an improvement of caecal motility.
- Cisapride (Prepulsid, Janssen UK Ltd.) is another motility drug and can be given at a dose of 0.5–1 mg/kg every 8–24 hours.

- The caecal flora should either be re-established permanently by transfaunation, or temporarily protected with *Lactobacillus* in a probiotic.

Prevention: The provision of a high fibre diet, and a gradual introduction to the pelleted ration at weaning. A probiotic such as Avipro (Vetark Health) can be dissolved in the drinking water at this vulnerable time. The use of tetracyclines at a concentration of 250 mg/litre in the drinking water for the first 10 days after weaning has been reported.

Comment: The aetiology of mucoid enteropathy is unclear, but recent work suggests that a dysautonomia (equivalent to 'grass sickness' in horses) may be responsible for the caecal paresis that triggers caecal dysbiosis.

Enterotoxaemia

- Affects rabbits of any age.

This describes the harmful consequence of the normal balance of micro-organisms in the caecum becoming disturbed. The balance tips in favour of harmful micro-organisms (*Clostridium spiriformes*). These bacteria multiply rapidly, producing endotoxins (iotatoxins) which cause rapid dehydration, collapse and death.
  Factors which lead to *Clostridium* proliferation are the following:

- An alteration in the caecal pH: normal pH is 5.9–6.8. If excess fermentable carbohydrates are fed, the caecum becomes more acidic and favours clostridial multiplication.
- A falling fibre content of the diet leads to a rise in populations of *E. coli* and *Clostridium*. Low fibre diets lead to a fall in volatile fatty acid production, and a rise in pH which unbalances the microflora.
- Oral administration of antibiotics (and to a lesser extent injectable antibiotics) will alter the normal balance of microflora.
- Excess dietary protein will lead to ammonia production in the caecum which will destabilise the caecal flora.
- Stress of any kind, e.g. weaning, a change of environment, hypothermia, will cause the release of adrenaline. This reduces gut motility and caecotroph production, which predisposes to *Clostridium* proliferation.
- Poor sanitation

Clinical signs: Anorexia and depression. Initially there is diarrhoea which is brown, watery and may contain blood or mucus. The rabbit soon becomes hypothermic and moribund. Death occurs within 24–48 hours. Some cases may become anorexic, bloat and die before diarrhoea develops. The abdomen sounds full of fluid if the rabbit is moved.

Diagnosis: Diagnosis is based on the history and clinical signs. At postmortem there may be haemorrhages on the serosal surface of the caecum, and haemorrhages and mucus present on the mucosal surface of the caecum and proximal colon. Gut stasis leads to the accumulation of gas throughout the digestive tract.

Treatment: The prognosis of these cases is guarded. Aggressive fluid therapy is essential. Metronidazole at a dose rate of 20 mg/kg orally twice daily may be of benefit. Repopulation of the intestinal flora can be achieved temporarily with a probiotic, or more permanently by transfaunation.

Vitamin C (ascorbic acid) may inhibit toxin production, and can be given at a dose of 50–100 mg/kg daily.

Cholestyramine (Questran, Bristol-Myers Pharmaceuticals Ltd.) can be given orally at a dose of 0.5 g/kg twice a day. This is an ion exchange resin that can bind the iotatoxins.

Prevention: The feeding of a high fibre hay-based diet is extremely important, particularly at any stressful or vulnerable time. The concentrated food should be rationed to prevent protein and carbohydrate overload. Vitamin C and a probiotic can be given at times of stress.

The use of a sheep vaccine (Covexin 8, Schering Plough Animal Health) has been reported in an outbreak of *Clostridium perfringens*. Two doses of 0.25 ml were given by subcutaneous injection 6 weeks apart and were successful in controlling the spread of the disease.

Colibacillosis in older rabbits

* Affects rabbits of any age post-weaning.

This disease can occur in rabbitries where there is poor husbandry and sanitation. It can also be a problem associated with pet shops where young rabbits from several sources may be mixed together.

Clinical signs: These depend upon the strain of *E. coli* involved, and range from a mild diarrhoea and weight loss, to a severe form of diarrhoea associated with up to 50% mortality.

Affected rabbits may develop an intussusception or rectal prolapse. Recovered animals may remain undersized.

Diagnosis: Isolation of *E. coli* from stool or tissue samples may suggest colibacillosis; however, non-pathogenic *E. coli* can be isolated from any rabbit, and in greater numbers from a rabbit with caecal dysbiosis. At post-mortem classic 'paintbrush' haemorrhages may be seen on the caecal wall. The colon will also be affected.

Treatment: Antibiotics (either trimethoprim–sulpha combinations or neomycin) fluids and a probiotic should be used. The fibre content of the diet should be increased.

Enterocolitis syndrome

This is a new disease condition first identified in France in 1997, and possibly seen in Belgium, Spain and Portugal. The syndrome was first seen in young rabbits of 5–7 weeks of age, but has also been reported in weanlings and lactating does. The disease appears to be highly contagious, and although the exact cause has not been identified it is thought it may be associated with a viral infection.

Clinical signs: Anorexia, a watery diarrhoea which is not profuse, reduced gastric motility progressing to ileus and death after 2–3 days. At post-mortem there is abundant liquid in the small intestine, and gas and mucus in the colon.

Tyzzer's disease

- Affects rabbits of any age. Not common in pet rabbits.

This is caused by *Clostridium piliforme* (formerly *Bacillus piliformis*). Other rodents are affected, and wild vermin may act as carriers of the disease. Any form of stress increases the rabbit's susceptibility to infection.

Clinical signs: Symptoms may be acute in the young rabbit. Signs include watery diarrhoea, listlessness, dehydration, anorexia and death. Older rabbits may develop chronic weight loss.

Diagnosis: At post-mortem there may be the classical focal necrosis of the liver, however, this is a less common finding than in other rodents. Silver staining of these lesions will identify the bacterium. The myocardium and gastrointestinal tract may have similar areas of necrosis. There may be oedema of the intestinal walls, especially in the caecum.

Treatment: There is a poor response to antibiotic therapy. Tetracyclines are the antibiotic of choice, and these can be given in the drinking water during an outbreak at a concentration of 125 mg/litre for up to a month.

Prevention: This is most important: stress should be minimised, and the rabbits should be fed on a high fibre (hay) diet. Wild rodents should be prevented from entering the environment, or contaminating the food. The bacterial spores will be killed by a 0.3% sodium hypochlorite solution.

Salmonellosis

This is uncommon, but can occur in association with contaminated food or water. It is generally caused by *Salmonella typhimurium*.

Clinical signs: Septicaemia, depression, pyrexia and death, often accompanied by diarrhoea.
   Does may develop metritis, and pregnant does may abort their young.

Diagnosis: Post-mortem findings reflect the septicaemia, diffuse petechial haemorrhages, and vascular congestion of organs. Necrotic foci are found on the liver and spleen. The lymph nodes may be oedematous.

Treatment: None. The disease is a zoonosis. Because of the public health risk affected animals should be destroyed, bedding and hay should be burnt, and all utensils thoroughly disinfected.

Miscellaneous bacteria

Diarrhoea associated with *Pseudomonas* has been reported in association with contamination of the drinkers.
   A *Campylobacter*-like organism has also been reported.

Enteritis complex

- Affects older rabbits.

Older rabbits can also show symptoms similar to the mucoid enteritis of young rabbits. The clinical signs may range from an intermittent diarrhoea, with stools covered in mucus, to a more severe diarrhoea which precipitates enterotoxaemia. Excess mucus is formed by both the caecal and colonic lumen.
   Any changes which upset the balance of the caecal flora can be

responsible for triggering this condition. Thus sudden dietary changes, stress, antibiosis or gut stasis can cause enteritis.

Treatment: This depends on the severity of the condition. Mild cases can be corrected by dietary changes such as increasing the fibre and decreasing the carbohydrate and protein content of the diet. More severe cases may need the same treatment as for mucoid enteropathy.

Antibiotic-induced diarrhoea

Oral administration of antibiotics, and to a lesser extent injectable antibiotics can alter the normal flora of the gastrointestinal tract, and allow *Clostridium* spp. to proliferate, causing enterotoxaemia. The most toxic drugs are those with a narrow spectrum of action against Gram-positive organisms such as penicillin, erythromycin, lincomycin and clindamycin. The negative effects of any antibiotic should be minimised by the concurrent use of a probiotic, and by ensuring that the rabbit is on a hay-rich high fibre diet.

Chronic diarrhoea

Some rabbits may present with diarrhoea of several months' duration. This must be differentiated from the build up of excess caecotrophs. There may be no hard pellets produced, and the liquid faeces will not have the strong smell that caecotrophs have.

Treatment: The diet should be changed to hay and astringent plants alone. All pelleted food and treats should be removed. Probiotics are particularly useful. Either Prozyme (Vetquimol UK Ltd.) or Avipro (Vetark Health) can be used. The recommended dose of Prozyme is $\frac{1}{4}$ teaspoon per cup of food. It is best to start with a lower dose and gradually increase it until the diarrhoea stops, as too much Prozyme may cause the rabbit to stop eating its caecal faeces and end up with 'sticky-bottom' syndrome.

Dietary enteritis

Any sudden change in diet can cause enteritis. Overfeeding can also cause enteritis. The 'carbohydrate overload theory' suggests that if there is too much grain starch in the diet the digestive capacity of the stomach and small intestine is exceeded, and undigested starch reaches the caecum, where it can alter the caecal pH, upset the microflora, and cause enteritis.

Diets and treats made with starch and refined sugars will have the same effect.

If large balls of concentrated foodstuffs enter the stomach they may not be effectively sterilised, allowing potentially harmful bacteria to enter the hind-gut.

Treatment: Provision of fibre is very important, and up to 20% of the diet should consist of coarse fibre. The rabbit should be provided with good hay only, plenty of fluids (given orally, or via subcutaneous injection), and the balance of microflora re-established, either with a probiotic, or by trans-faunation. Astringent plants can be introduced to the diet before re-introducing the dry food.

VIRAL DISEASES

Rotavirus

Infection with rotavirus alone may be subclinical, and it may be endemic in some situations. However, in association with stress and secondary infection it can produce severe clinical signs of anorexia, diarrhoea, dehydration and death. Suckling and weanling rabbits between 4 and 12 weeks of age are most vulnerable.

Pathology: There is villous atrophy of the jejunum and ileum. The intestines are distended and congested, and there are petechial haemorrhages in the small and large intestines.

Diagnosis: This is by virus isolation.

Prevention: This is difficult as the virus may be endemic. Stress of all forms should be reduced, and the diet should be improved to include more fibre in the form of hay.

Coronavirus

A coronavirus has been identified that causes disease in rabbits between 3 and 10 weeks of age. In this age group the clinical signs are severe anorexia, diarrhoea, dehydration and death, whilst adult rabbits can carry the virus subclinically.

Pathology: This is similar to that produced by a rotavirus.

Diagnosis: This is via virus isolation.

Calicivirus

Viral haemorrhagic disease is caused by a calicivirus (see Chapter 14).

ENDOPARASITES

Stomach worm

This is found in wild rabbits, and occasionally in pet rabbits. The worms (*Graphidium strigosum*) are red, 1–2 cm long, and found on the stomach lining. In large numbers they may cause weight loss and death.

Treatment: A roundworm product such as fenbendazole (Panacur, Hoechst UK Ltd.) can be used at a dose of 10–20 mg/kg orally. Ivermectin given by subcutaneous injection at a dose of 0.4 mg/kg is also effective.

Pinworm

These worms (*Passalurus ambiguous*) are thought to be non-pathogenic. They are very small (0.5 cm long) and found in the rectum and stuck by the anus. They have a direct life-cycle; the adults live in the caecum and colon, and eggs are passed in the faeces.

Treatment: Fenbendazole (Panacur, Hoechst UK Ltd.) can be used at a dose of 10–20 mg/kg orally, and repeated in 14 days. Treatment is not strictly necessary as the worms are non-pathogenic, but owners may prefer not to see them. Ivermectin is also effective against pinworms at a dose of 0.4 mg/kg.

Tapeworm

These are considered to be very rare. The rabbit is the definitive host of *Mosgovoyia pectinata*, the adult stage of which is found in the small intestine, and segments of which are passed in the faeces. The eggs from the segments are eaten by free living mites in which the worm embryo develops. Mites containing the infective larval stage are then ingested by rabbits as they graze.

The rabbit is also an intermediate host for *Taenia pisiformis* and *Taenia serialis*. The dog is the definitive host for these tapeworms, and the rabbit can become infected if it grazes on vegetation soiled by dog faeces. The intermediate stages can be found in infected rabbits: cysticerci in the liver and mesentery, and coenuri in the muscle and connective tissue.

Treatment: Praziquantel (Droncit, Bayer AG) can be given by sub-cutaneous injection at a dose of 5–10 mg/kg. This can be repeated after 10 days.

Coccidiosis

Coccidia are the commonest parasites of the rabbit. Twelve forms of this protozoal parasite are known to infect the rabbit, all from the genus *Eimeria*. One species, *Eimeria stiedai* parasitises the liver, whilst the rest colonise the gastrointestinal tract. Not all species are pathogenic. The most common intestinal species are *Eimeria perforans*, *Eimeria magna* and *Eimeria media*.

Hepatic coccidiosis

This is caused by *Eimeria stiedae*. The parasite colonises the biliary epithelium, and the oocytes produced pass down the bile duct and into the faeces. Sporulation requires 2 days or more outside the host. Infection is spread via the faeco-oral route, by ingestion of sporulated oocysts. Caecotrophs, however, are not part of this cycle as caecotrophy does not allow time for sporulation and the caecotrophs never contain oocysts.

Clinical signs: In mild infections young rabbits may just show general unthriftiness, or the disease may be fatal. Heavily infected rabbits show symptoms associated with bile duct blockage, an enlarged and failing liver, ascites, jaundice, diarrhoea, anorexia and death.

Diagnosis: The presence of coccidial oocysts does not always confirm the diagnosis, as many rabbits are subclinically infected with coccidia. However, the isolation of large numbers of coccidia, and the presence of clinical signs will suggest coccidiosis.

At post-mortem the liver is enlarged and covered with yellow–white nodules. When these nodules are cut they exude a yellow–green fluid. The same fluid may be found in the gall bladder and bile duct. The number of foci is related to the number of infected oocysts ingested. Histopathological examination of the liver will confirm the diagnosis.

Treatment: In large rabbitries, pellets may be fed that contain a cocci-diostat. However, strains of coccidia can become resistant to these drugs;

they also appear less effective against hepatic than intestinal coccidia. Sulpha drugs are the most effective.

Sulphadimidine (Intradine, Norbrook Laboratories Ltd.) can be given in the drinking water at a concentration of 0.2%. To achieve this concentration 1 ml of Sulphamezathine 33% can be diluted in 150 ml water (i.e. 6 ml/litre). This can be given as three 3 day courses, with two 2 day intervals in between.

Sulphadimethoxine can be given orally at a dose of 25 mg/kg daily for 10–14 days.

Alternatively a trimethoprim–sulpha combination can be given by mouth at a dose of 30 mg/kg twice daily. The combined amount of trimethoprim and sulpha drug is used when working out the dose rate. The treatment should be continued for 10–14 days.

Amprolium 9.6% in the drinking water is also effective.

Attention to hutch sanitation is extremely important because the oocysts thrive in damp conditions. Hutches should be cleaned and disinfected regularly, as the oocysts can remain infectious in the environment for several months.

Intestinal coccidiosis

The life cycle of these *Eimeria* species is similar to *Eimeria stiedae*, except that the ingested oocysts colonise the intestines. The site and pathogenicity depend upon the species. *Eimeria magna* is highly pathogenic of the small intestine, *Eimeria perforans* is of low pathogenicity of the small intestine, and *Eimeria media* is of moderate pathogenicity of both large and small intestines. Mixed infections are common.

Clinical signs: These depend upon the species, and on the quantity of infective oocysts that are ingested. Mild infections are unapparent, and a previous exposure leads to the development of immunity. Clinical signs are most common in young rabbits, and include diarrhoea, weight loss, anorexia and, in severe cases, dehydration and death due to secondary bacteraemia. The diarrhoea frequently contains blood and mucus. If the diarrhoea is severe it may lead to the development of intussusception.

Diagnosis: Oocysts will be found on faecal examination; however, oocysts can also be found in healthy rabbits, so results must be interpreted with care. At post-mortem there are ulcerative lesions of the intestinal lumen. Definitive diagnosis is by histopathological examination of the intestines.

Treatment: See Hepatic coccidiosis.

Prevention of coccidiosis: Elimination of coccidia is difficult, as many rabbits may develop an immunity following previous exposure and become carriers, particularly in the case of hepatic coccidiosis. Attention to hutch sanitation is most important. The oocysts need at least 2 days in the environment to sporulate and become infective, and they thrive in damp conditions; therefore regular cleaning of the hutch will remove these oocysts. As oocysts can survive for many months in the environment, deep-litter situations are not recommended, and if the rabbit is kept in an ark on the grass it should be moved regularly.

   Stress of any sort such as overcrowding or poor nutrition make rabbits more susceptible to clinical disease, and any stress factors must be reduced.

Yeasts

The yeast *Saccharomyces* is a normal inhabitant of the caecum. The numbers of this yeast vary with the composition of the diet; as the fibre content of the diet increases the number of *Saccharomyces* falls.

ANOREXIA

This may be associated with pain of any sort or stress. A full clinical examination is essential to determine the cause of the problem, and the following treatment protocol can be instigated whilst investigations are underway.

   The aim of treatment is to provide enough calories to prevent hepatic lipidosis, to rehydrate the gastrointestinal contents, and to provide indigestible fibre to help promote peristalsis.

Treatment:

- Keep the rabbit in an environmental temperature of less than 24°C (75°F).
- Fluid replacement. Lactated Ringer's solution (Hartmann's solution) can be given by subcutaneous injection at 100 ml/kg per day.
- Analgesics.
- Offer leafy greens, dandelions, parsley, carrot tops, or kale immediately. Fresh hay should also be available.
- Syringe feeding. A mixture of pineapple juice, ground pellets and strained vegetable baby food in a 1:1:1 ratio can be given. 10–15 ml/kg of this mixture can be fed two or three times a day. Canned pumpkin

and alfalfa powder, if available, can be added to the mixture. V-8 vegetable juice (Campbells) can be included in the mixture instead of pineapple juice. The mixture should be made fresh daily, as if left for longer it will ferment. Force feeding is very important to correct or prevent hepatic lipidosis which occurs very quickly after a rabbit stops eating. If necessary the rabbit should be fed through a nasogastric tube.

- Metoclopramide can be given at a dose of 0.5 mg/kg up to four times daily to stimulate normal gut motility.
- Vitamin C 50–100 mg/kg twice daily, together with vitamin B (1–2 mg/ kg thiamine) if caecotrophy is impaired; in the latter case Multivet 4BC injection (C-Vet) can be given at a dose of 0.3 ml/kg.
- Antibiotic therapy may be given if indicated. Enrofloxacin or a tri-methoprim–sulpha combination are safest. The latter can help protect against caecal dysbiosis.
- A probiotic such as Avipro (Vetark Health) will help prevent caecal dysbiosis.

LEAD POISONING

This is included here as it should be in the differential diagnosis for anorexia, particularly since more rabbits are kept free range indoors with potential access to lead in old paint, curtain weights, the foil around wine bottles, etc.

Clinical signs: These may be vague and include anorexia, lethargy and neurological changes. Anorexia and weight loss are the most common symptoms.

Diagnosis: An abdominal radiograph may show ingested metal in the abdomen. A blood sample for lead levels should be taken, and haematology may reveal basophilic stippling of the red blood cells.

Treatment: Rabbits with a blood lead level greater than 10 µg/dL should be treated with injections of calcium versenate (Ca-EDTA). The dose is 27.5 mg/kg by subcutaneous injection four times a day for 5 days. A second course may be required a week later.

USE OF A NASOGASTRIC TUBE

This can be used for rabbits that are debilitated, or those that cannot tolerate force feeding or oral medications. The tube can be left in place for several weeks if necessary, and until the rabbit starts eating of its own accord. Rabbits can eat whilst a nasogastric tube is in position. A 5–8 Fr (1.6–2.6 mm diameter) tube should be used, and be measured and marked against the side of the rabbit before it is used. A little local anaesthetic can be placed into the nostril and the tube should be lubricated with some local anaesthetic gel. The tube should be placed in the ventral meatus and gently directed ventrally and medially.

The correct positioning of the tube must be checked by radiograph, as rabbits may not cough when fluids are unintentionally passed into the chest. The tube can then be taped to the bridge of the nose and the top of the head. If necessary a tab can be made with sticking plaster around the end of the tube, and this can be sutured to the skin at the top of the head. Most rabbits will tolerate a tube, but some may need to wear an Elizabethan collar to prevent them dislodging the tube with their feet.

The nasogastric tube can be used to give oral medication, and nutritional support. A solution of soaked rabbit pellets and puréed vegetables can be given at a rate of 10–15 ml/kg two or three times daily. A probiotic and vitamins can be added to this mixture. The tube should be flushed with water before and after every feeding or medication.

OBESITY

Clinical significance:

- Hepatic lipidosis
- Pododermatitis (see Chapter 4)
- Chronic soft stools

Obesity is a real problem in pet rabbits. Most rabbits are fed a diet rich in carbohydrates and protein, and given extra treats, whilst getting little or no exercise. The key to managing obesity is to make gradual changes. The diet should be based on hay and leafy green foods, with no or little dry food. If the rabbit is already used to eating hay, the dry food can be removed completely; otherwise it should be removed gradually whilst the rabbit becomes accustomed to the hay and greens. If food intake declines rapidly the rabbit may develop hepatic lipidosis. A gradual weight loss of no more than 1–2% of the body weight per week should be the recommended target.

THE LIVER

Normal biochemical parameters

- ALT (alanine aminotransferase): 22–80 iu/litre
- ALKP (alkaline phosphatase): 15–90 iu/litre
- AST (aspartate aminotransferase): 14–113 iu/litre
- BUN (blood area nitrogen): 17–24 mg/dl (6.06–6.56 mmol/litre)
- GGT (γ-glutamyltransferase): 0–7 iu/litre
- Total protein: 5.4–7.5 g/dl (54–75 g/litre)

ALT is the most sensitive marker of hepatocellular damage. ALKP also occurs in the intestinal epithelium, renal tubules and osteoblasts, and young rabbits normally have levels 2–4 times greater than adults.

AST is used to diagnose liver and muscle disease and increases are associated with liver cell necrosis.

GGT is found mainly in the biliary epithelium, and an increase will indicate post-hepatic liver damage. It does not increase following hepato-cellular damage.

BUN will be reduced in severe hepatic insufficiency.

Total protein, in particular albumin (normally 60% of the total protein) will be reduced in both liver and renal disease.

Hepatic lipidosis

The rabbit is very susceptible to the development of hepatic lipidosis. Even a short period of anorexia will lead to ketosis, and subsequent hepatic lipidosis. Ketonuria can be detected by the use of urine test strips. Liver biochemical parameters will be elevated.

Treatment: Rehydration with glucose–saline or lactated Ringer's solution (Hartmann's solution). If the rabbit is anorexic, force feeding is essential to maintain a positive energy balance.

Hepatic insufficiency

Pine and cedar shavings can cause liver disease. The removal of these from the litter tray will usually allow for a reversal of the condition to occur.

Liver biochemical parameters will be raised; however, in severe hepatic insufficiency the BUN will be decreased, and the total protein will also be lowered.

THE SPLEEN

Yersiniosis

An enlarged spleen may be caused by infection with *Yersinia pseudotuberculosis* (rodentosis). Clinical signs are non-specific and include cachexia and weight loss. The spleen is palpable on clinical examination.

The bacterium is carried by rodents and birds, and is introduced to the rabbitry by contamination of food and bedding, and from the feeding of unwashed plants. Prevention is therefore aimed at controlling rodents and washing fresh feedstuffs.

Diagnosis of yersiniosis is not possible in the live rabbit. Post-mortem examination of infected rabbits reveals the enlarged spleen with necrotic foci on its surface, and similar foci in the lymphoid tissue at the ileo-caecal junction. The bacteria can be isolated from these foci. If yersiniosis is suspected in the live rabbit, treatment can be attempted with enrofloxacin at a dose of 5 mg/kg twice daily for 3–4 weeks.

Salmonellosis

In acute salmonellosis (see page 94) the spleen may be enlarged tenfold. Pathology reveals necrotic foci on the spleen, liver and Peyer's patches. There may be an associated metritis.

Toxoplasmosis

Splenomegaly is also seen in acute toxoplasmosis. The cat is the definitive host for the protozoan *Toxoplasma gondii*, and infection occurs if the rabbit eats food that is contaminated with cat faeces carrying the oocyst stage. Chronic infections remain unapparent, but the acute form causes anorexia, lethargy, fever, tremors, muscle weakness and paralysis.

To avoid infection occurring, cats must be kept away from the rabbit's environment.

THE PANCREAS

Normal biochemical parameters

- α-Amylase: 200–500 iu/litre. α-Amylase is found in high concentrations in the pancreas, and increased levels are found in pancreatic obstruction and damage to the exocrine tissue of the pancreas.

- Blood glucose: 75–150 g/dl (4.2–8.3 mmol/l)

Diabetes is not generally considered as a clinical disease in rabbits, although it has been reported in New Zealand White rabbits. Experimentally rabbits have been shown to survive following a pancreactomy, suggesting that the role of the pancreas is not as important as in other mammals.

Detection of glucose in the urine is a normal finding, and a raised blood glucose does not necessarily imply a diagnosis of diabetes as it may occur with excitement, hyperthermia, shock and in early mucoid enteritis.

Rabbits that have a persistently raised blood glucose and are polydipsic can be managed on a hay-based high fibre diet. If the rabbit is obese the dry food can be cut out of the daily ration.

NEOPLASIA OF THE GASTROINTESTINAL TRACT

Various neoplasms have been identified. They may be primary lesions, or secondaries (generally from uterine adenocarcinomas). Some neoplasms may be amenable to surgical resection if identified early. Bile duct carcinomas are the exception as metastasis is common.

- Stomach: adenocarcinoma, leiomyosarcoma
- Intestines: leiomyoma, leiomyosacoma
- Sacculus rotundus: papilloma
- Bile duct: adenoma, carcinoma
- Rectum: anorectal papilloma

Lymphosarcoma

This is the second most common neoplasm of the rabbit, and it generally affects visceral rather than peripheral lymph nodes. The liver, spleen, kidneys and bone marrow become affected. Clinical signs include lethargy, anorexia, anaemia and weight loss. The prognosis is poor.

SURGERY OF THE GASTROINTESTINAL TRACT

Surgery may be necessary in cases of gastric impaction, foreign body ingestion, intussusception, or neoplasia. The quality of post-surgical nursing must be high to give the rabbit patient the best chance of recovery after surgery. The rabbit should be maintained in a warm environment, and force fed until it starts eating again to prevent the development of hepatic lipidosis. Fluids and soft foods only should be given for the first 48 hours whilst any gastrointestinal incisions are healing. Probiotics should be given to prevent stress-induced dysbiosis.

Gastrotomy

This procedure should only be considered if medical management with fluids and gastrointestinal motility drugs have failed to improve motility after 3–4 days of therapy. A midline incision is made so that the stomach can be visualised, and the stomach is exteriorised and packed off with moist swabs to prevent contamination of the abdomen with stomach contents. The gastrotomy incision is made in the avascular section between lesser and greater curvatures. The gastric impaction is generally a felt of hair and fibrous food entwined together, and can often be removed as one large single mass. The gastrotomy wound should be closed in two layers with 1.5–2 metric chromic catgut, using a continuous inverting pattern that extends into, but not through, the gastric mucosa.

The abdomen should be lavaged with saline at body temperature before closure.

Enterotomy and intestinal resection

This procedure may be necessary in cases of foreign body ingestion, and intussusception. A midline abdominal incision is made to visualise the gastrointestinal contents. The affected portions of intestine should be isolated with non-crushing bowel clamps. The bowel should be exteriorised from the abdomen and packed with soaked swabs to prevent accidental contamination of the abdomen with intestinal contents. Enterotomy wounds may be best made longitudinally, and then closed transversely if the bowel diameter is small, and can be sutured with 1.5–2 metric chromic catgut with simple interrupted apposition sutures. Inverting sutures should not be used as they will further narrow the diameter of the lumen.

If a resection is necessary, care must be taken to preserve as much of the vasculature as possible. The intestine can be cut at an angle, so that the diameter of the lumen at the site of anastomosis is as wide as possible. The anastomosis can be performed using 1.5 metric chromic catgut using a simple interrupted appositional suture.

Large bowel surgery

This is rarely done: the mucosal wall is very thin and tears easily. Incisions in the colon wall can be sutured with an apposition suture, whereas the wall of the caecum can be closed with a continuous inverting suture.

10   THE MUSCULOSKELETAL SYSTEM

THE SKELETON

The rabbit skeleton is fragile compared with those of other mammals, representing only 7–8% of the total body mass. Rabbits can easily fracture bones or break their backs if they struggle when restrained. House rabbits that have opportunity to exercise, and to build up bone and muscle strength are less susceptible to spinal injuries.

Toenails

The rabbit has five digits on the forelegs, and four digits on the hind legs. Each digit has a toenail, with a central quick. When clipping the nail it is important to cut below the quick to avoid bleeding. Rabbits commonly pull out their nails when they struggle, and the quicks may bleed profusely. If a nail is lost, the nail bed must be kept clean and antibiotics given when necessary. Any bleeding can be cauterised using potassium permanganate, and a dressing can be applied. The development of a nail bed infection will cause the swelling of the affected digit, and if untreated may progress to osteomyelitis.

Pododermatitis (sore hocks)

Clinical signs: Hair loss, scaling, erythema and ulceration of the skin on the plantar aspect of the metatarsus. Very occasionally the front feet may be affected too. The development of this condition is associated with abrasive or soiled cage floors, in conjunction with obesity and in rabbits that stamp frequently. In house rabbits it may be associated with 'carpet-burn'. It is common in rabbits that only have a thin covering of fur on the foot pad.

The lesions become secondarily infected with *Pasteurella multocida* or *Staphylococcus aureus*, and may develop caseous abscesses. Occasionally the condition may progress to cause osteomyelitis and septicaemia.

Treatment: The lesions should be cleaned with an antiseptic such as povidone–iodine, or Clenderm (Univet Ltd.). Dermisol (Pfizer Ltd.) or Clenderm cream can be applied topically several times a day. Both Clenderm and Dermisol contain (Pfizer Ltd.) propylene glycol, organic acids and salicylic acid. If the rabbit will tolerate dressings, the feet may be dressed. Dressings should be changed every 5 days, and once the hock is healing the area can be protected with a lighter covering such as a small sock. A soft, clean surface (either deep dry bedding or towels) should be provided.

The injection of a long-acting steroid under the lesion may be of benefit. The lesions can take weeks to heal.

A tendency towards sore hocks may be inherited, and affected animals should not be bred from. Owners should be advised not to trim the fur pads from the point of the hock, but rather to wash the hocks in warm water, as fur trimming, especially in Angoras can predispose towards sore hocks.

Fractures

Rabbits readily fracture their legs. Their habit of stamping with their hind legs, or kicking out when they struggle means that they are also susceptible to vertebral fractures, often in the region of L6–L7. Rabbits that are selective feeders, and may have a low calcium intake, are more susceptible to fractures. Diagnosis of fractures is by radiography.

Fracture repair

Fractured legs can be managed in the same way as for cats and dogs.

External fixation: The cast material must be light enough so that the rabbit is not hindered by the dressing. A half-cast and a light Robert Jones bandage may provide adequate support. Problems that may occur are the chewing of the dressing by the patient, or the dressing may become soiled, causing skin infections and pressure sores. Closed fractures should have a single dose of antibiotics at the time of stabilisation.

External fixators have also been used to repair fractures. These need to be left in place for at least 6 weeks. Antibiotics should be given post-operatively.

Internal fixation: Many fractures can be repaired with intramedullary pins. Great care must be taken to debride and lavage open fracture wounds, as post-traumatic osteomyelitis is a common complication of infected fracture sites. Fractures managed by internal fixation need post-operative antibiotics for 7–10 days.

Post-operative care

Whatever method is used for fracture fixation the post-operative care should be the same. Analgesia should be given at the time of stabilisation, and continued post-operatively as necessary. Post-operative antibiosis is important for open fractures to prevent the development of post-traumatic osteomyelitis.

The patient should be confined in a clean stress-free environment. Force feeding may be necessary if the rabbit is anorexic. Pain is often manifest as anorexia, so these patients should continue to receive analgesia.

The fracture should be re-radiographed every 3–4 weeks to monitor the healing process. Callus formation may take as little as 10 days, and healing of an uncomplicated fracture is generally complete by 6 weeks.

Post-traumatic osteomyelitis

This is a potential complication of an open fracture, if the fracture site is contaminated or the vascular supply is damaged. Open fractures must be debrided and lavaged before repair to try and prevent this condition. Post-operative antibiosis, preferably based on the results of a culture, are very important and should be given for 7–10 days, or longer if necessary.

Radiographic signs of post-traumatic osteomyelitis include osteolysis and periosteal reactions around the fracture site. An abscess may develop at the fracture site, often associated with *Pseudomonas* infection. Treatment with further antibiotics and wound lavage is generally unsuccessful, and amputation of the limb may be the only solution.

Osteomyelitis

Bacterial infection of bone can occur in the jaw, commonly associated with tooth root abscesses, and in the long bones secondary to pododermatitis, or nail-bed infections. Radiographically there is osteolysis and secondary new bone production associated with the area of infection. There may be drainage tracts in the bone associated with severe osteomyelitis.

Osteomyelitis is very difficult to treat, and requires surgical debridement of the affected area and the use of long-term antibiotics. Local impregnation of the affected area with antibiotics can be attempted. Where a limb is affected amputation may be necessary.

Amputation

Rabbits cope extremely well with the loss of a limb, either a fore or hind leg. The procedure for amputation is similar to that for a cat or dog. The forelimb is best amputated through the proximal humerus, whilst preserving as much muscle bulk as possible. The hind leg can be amputated at the proximal femur, whilst preserving the bulk of the quadriceps muscle. In smaller rabbits which may be lightly muscled, the femur is best removed at the coxo-femoral joint. Similarly if the hind limb is being amputated to resolve a congenitally dislocated hip, it can be removed at the coxo-femoral joint. Care must be taken when cutting the bones, as they can shatter easily, and are better cut with a rotating saw than bone-cutters. The muscle edges are inverted and sewn with a continuous suture using chromic cat gut, and skin closure is done with a continuous apposition suture. A single dose of post-operative antibiotics is necessary, and analgesia should be given for the first 24–48 hours.

Spinal cord injury

Traumatic vertebral injury with spinal cord damage commonly occurs in pet rabbits. The onset is acute and it may occur even after a slight struggle.

Radiographs are necessary to assess the injury. Spinal fractures occur most commonly at L6 and L7. The prognosis depends upon the degree of spinal cord damage.

Spinal cord injury in the absence of a vertebral fracture results in oedema around the cord. The rabbit should be given a rapid acting corticosteroid, and diuretics, and be cage rested. If some motor function to the hind limbs and bladder are retained at the time of injury, the prognosis for recovery is good.

Nursing a rabbit with paresis or paralysis is very important. Food and water must be accessible, and the rabbit may need to be supported in a sitting position whilst it eats. The main complication is urinary and faecal soiling. The rabbit may need to be bathed regularly using a mild solution of chlorhexidine. The perineal area can be protected from urine scald by the use of a resistant barrier cream such as zinc and castor oil cream, or kept dry with the application of baby talcum powder. If urinary incontinence is a problem the rabbit can wear disposable nappies, or be bedded on an absorbent material such as 'Vetbed' or sheepskin. Care must be taken to avoid myiasis ('fly strike') if there is perineal soiling.

Rabbits with spinal cord paresis will be unable to practice coprophagy. They should therefore be given a vitamin supplement, and weekly vitamin B injections. The caecotrophs they produce can be collected, and be fed back to them.

Geriatric rabbits can develop paresis and paralysis as a result of vertebral degeneration in association with ageing, and vertebral spondylosis is common. These rabbits should be nursed as above. Anti-inflammatory treatment can be given on a daily basis, and some patients may respond to complementary medicine such as acupuncture.

Arthritis

Reduced mobility in the older rabbit may be associated with arthritis. Radiographs will show marked periosteal proliferation in cases of degenerative joint disease. There may be associated soft tissue calcification or ossification.

Analgesia can be given to control the pain. Aspirin as a paediatric syrup can be given at a dose of 100 mg/kg twice daily. Meloxicam (Metacam, Boehringer Ingelheim Ltd.) can be also be given in liquid form. Long term corticosteroid use is contraindicated as it may activate subclinical *Pasteurella* infection. Complementary therapies such as acupuncture may be of benefit. If mobility is limited, the rabbit will be more prone to urinary and faecal soiling, and can be bedded on a soft absorbent bedding such as 'Vetbed'. Food and water should be made easily available, and a litter tray, if used, should have a low or absent rim so that it is easily accessible. If the rabbit is overweight it should be encouraged to lose weight slowly, by reducing its concentrate ration, and introducing more hay and greens.

Osteoporosis

This is a metabolic bone disease which results from diets that are too low in calcium. Rabbits can become selective feeders and those that leave the pelleted portion of their dry mix (which contains the calcium and vitamins) are most at risk. Lack of exercise can predispose to osteoporosis.

Radiographically there is a decreased skeletal radiodensity. Radiographs of the spine will show indistinct transverse and dorsal spinous processes, and the vertebral end plates will be less dense than the vertebral bodies.

Rabbits with osteoporosis are more prone to vertebral injury, and also dental malocclusion, as the poor mineralisation of the periodontal bone allows tooth movement in the sockets, and therefore malocclusion.

Rabbits should be made to eat all parts of a complete ration. Less should be given, and the bowl should not be topped up until it is finished. A vitamin and mineral supplement, e.g. Arkvits (VetArk), can be sprinkled on the food. Rabbits should be allowed a minimum of 4 hours exercise a day.

Neoplasia

Osteosarcomas are generally found in the jaw bones, where they should be differentiated from osteomyelitis by radiography. Osteosarcomas have also been recorded on other parts of the appendicular skeleton.

Osteochondromas are found on the long bones of the skeleton.

Neoplasia carries a very poor prognosis.

Conditions of young rabbits

Splay leg

This is a congenital condition and is noticed when the young begin to leave the nest. One or more limbs are spread out, and the rabbit is unable to move properly. Splayed legs can result from femoral luxation or subluxation, distal foreleg curvature, or achondroplasia of the hip or shoulder. There is generally no cure, and euthanasia may the only option. Kits with only one affected limb may be able to manage until they are old enough to undergo amputation of the affected limb, which will greatly increase their overall mobility.

Hind leg paresis

This can occur spontaneously in rabbits of 12–14 weeks of age. The hind legs are weak and proprioception and withdrawal reflexes are reduced or absent. The administration of anti-inflammatory drugs, and the oral dosing of tomato juice (a rich source of potassium) appear to resolve the condition in many cases.

Musculodystrophy and hind leg paralysis

These can be seen in association with vitamin E deficiency and can also occur in older rabbits. There is marked skeletal muscle degeneration.

MUSCLE

Biochemical parameters

- AST (aspartate aminotransferase): 14–113 iu/litre
- CK (creatine kinase): 0.5–2.5 mg/dl (44–177 mmol/litre)

Both these enzymes are found in muscle and will be raised even with restraint. CK is a rapid and specific indicator of muscle degeneration. Dutch rabbits may develop higher levels of muscle enzymes as they appear to be more sensitive to trauma.

Myositis

A severe myositis is associated with sarcocystis. The causative agent is *Sarcocystis cuniculi*, which forms cysts in the skeletal muscle, particularly in the hind legs. Although the intact cysts cause no symptoms, when a cyst ruptures it causes myositis. The wild cottontail rabbit is a common host for *Sarcocystis*, and pet rabbits should be kept away from these rabbits. There is no cure for sarcocystis.

11   THE TEETH

INTRODUCTION

Rabbits have 28 teeth, all of which grow continuously throughout their life. They have two upper and two lower incisors, and two tiny teeth behind the upper incisors known as peg teeth. The function of the peg teeth is to prevent the lower incisors impinging on the upper gum. The incisors are designed for gnawing and may grow 10–12.5 cm (4–5 inches) in 1 year. There are 22 molars (the cheek teeth), six on the top and five on the bottom, both sides. The cheek teeth are designed for chewing, and the rabbit moves its jaw from side to side to wear these teeth evenly. Wild rabbits spend 3–4 hours every day chewing grass and plants, ensuring adequate wear of these teeth. Unfortunately the diet of the pet rabbit does not always provide enough to chew, and dry foods make the rabbit chew with a crushing action, rather than the desired sideways movement.

Rabbits have a set of deciduous teeth which are shed at the time of their birth, and their permanent teeth are fully erupted between 3 and 5 weeks of age.

MALOCCLUSION

The rabbit, like other rodents, has certain teeth peculiarities which make it prone to malocclusion, a situation where the teeth wear unevenly and become overgrown.

(1)   The teeth grow continually, and their state can be affected by changes in nutrition.
(2)   The teeth are hypsodontic: this means the crown of the tooth is bigger than the root.

(3) The jaw action for even wear of the teeth is both scissor (up and down) and from side to side.

(4) The shape of the skull may make certain breeds more susceptible to malocclusion. Short-nosed breeds such as the dwarf lops may be prone to incisor malocclusion, whereas narrow-faced breeds may suffer from molar malocclusion. This is presumably due to the differing jaw actions due to the difference in jaw configuration.

Malocclusion can either affect the front (incisor) teeth, or back (molar) teeth. In the author's experience it is generally one set of teeth or the other, rarely both. The only exception is when incisor overgrowth is so severe it hinders jaw movement, allowing subsequent overgrowth of the molars.

Incisor malocclusion

This condition occurs when the front teeth do not wear evenly, resulting in overgrowth of the teeth, which impairs eating. There are five main types of malocclusion, based on the reasons that it occurs (Harcourt Brown, 1997).

(1) *Congenital (hereditary) malocclusion*. This is most commonly seen in the short-nosed breeds such as the dwarf and lop eared breeds (mandibular prognathism).

(2) *Tooth root infection*. In these cases pus may be seen at the gum margins of the front teeth. Subsequent tooth pain and a reduction in appetite will lead to an overgrowth of the front teeth.

(3) *Tooth trauma*. The front teeth may be damaged by a fall, or may break on the cage bars. Damage to the teeth in this way may lead to malocclusion. Unfortunately teeth trimming, which is at present the common treatment for malocclusion, may traumatise the teeth further if they splinter when trimmed, and therefore perpetuate the problem.

(4) *Head trauma*. Although uncommon, this may occur after a dog or fox attack, causing jaw damage, non-alignment of the teeth, and subsequent malocclusion.

(5) *Primary molar malocclusion*. If the molars wear unevenly this will in turn cause the incisors to overgrow.

More recently a study by Harcourt-Brown (1997) has shown that poor bone and tooth quality due to calcium deficiency may play a primary role in the development of malocclusion. Calcium and vitamin D deficiency result in osteomalacia of the skull, so that the teeth move more freely in their sockets, and are of poor quality with defective enamel.

Clinical signs: Weight loss, dysphagia; the long incisors will be evident on clinical examination, often entwined with hair or food. The teeth may cause secondary damage to the gums which will become infected. The incisors may have horizontal ridges in their enamel indicating their poor quality.

Treatment: Classically the incisor teeth have been cut with nail clippers. However, this method can cause the teeth to splinter, predisposing the rabbit to tooth root infection, and worsening the malocclusion. It is recommended that the teeth are trimmed using a high speed dental burr or cutting disc. A mouth guard should be placed behind the teeth to protect the tongue. The teeth will need to be trimmed every 4–5 weeks due to their speed of regrowth.

Alternatively the incisors can be extracted, providing a permanent solution.

Procedure for incisor extraction

The rabbit should be sedated with an injectable combination. Xylazine and ketamine can be given in the same syringe by intramuscular injection. The dose is xylazine 5 mg/kg and ketamine 25 mg/kg. Other combinations of drugs are available (see Anaesthesia).

A lateral radiograph should be taken of the head to ascertain the degree of curvature of the upper incisors, and to look for the presence of osteomyelitis.

The upper incisors are removed first. The epithelial attachments surrounding the teeth are gently broken down with a specialist elevator or a 19 gauge needle. The teeth should be extracted following the curvature of the tooth. The peg teeth are then removed. The lower incisors are then removed in the same fashion. As the teeth are removed it is very important to disrupt any remaining dental pulp, as if any cells are left the teeth can regrow. This can be done by gently moving the incisor up and down in the socket before it is finally removed, or by moving a fine sterilised piece of metal in the socket after extraction. The top incisors are removed first so that if necessary the sedation can be topped up with some inhalation anaesthesia whilst the lower incisors are extracted.

Post-operative antibiotics should be given for 5–10 days to prevent infection in the tooth sockets. Analgesia should also be given at the time of surgery. After surgery the rabbit usually begins eating in 6–8 hours, often sooner. Initially shredded or grated food should be offered. A probiotic should also be given for the duration of the antibiotics and it will be a useful appetite stimulant.

Molar malocclusion

Molar malocclusion can develop for several reasons. There may be a breed tendency for it to develop, related to skull shape. Anything that interferes with normal tooth movement may lead to tooth overgrowth. Alterations in the consistency of the diet will lead to tooth overgrowth, refined diets do not provide enough for chewing; diets based on hay are beneficial. A tooth that becomes loose, either as a result of food impaction or infection will hinder normal jaw movement and lead to uneven wear and overgrowth. Incisor overgrowth will also hinder normal jaw action. The molars then wear unevenly, and spurs from the lower molars grow into the tongue, whilst spurs from the upper molars grow towards the cheek. The subsequent lingual and buccal ulceration is extremely painful.

Clinical signs: Weight loss, a reduced number of droppings, sticky bottoms (as the rabbit is no longer comfortable to eat its caecal faeces), difficulty chewing, and salivation. The medial aspect of each foreleg may be stained and damp as the rabbit paws at its mouth. An ocular discharge may also be present. Often anorexia is the only clinical sign, and molar malocclusion should be the first differential to consider in any anorexic rabbit. The mouth can be examined using a metal vaginal speculum, and a more detailed examination can be done under sedation, using special mouth gags and cheek dilators. Another indication of molar disease is the presence of hard swellings along the ventral borders of the mandible caused by periosteal penetration by the roots of the lower cheek teeth. As dental disease advances these roots may become the sites of facial abscesses.

Treatment: The rabbit is sedated with an injectable anaesthetic. Pouch dilators and gags will allow good visualisation of the cheek teeth, and any spurs can be trimmed and filed to restore the teeth to as near normal as possible. A low-speed straight dental burr can be used for this purpose, or diamond impregnated rabbit tooth rasps are also available. The crowns can be reduced to the gum if necessary. Post-operatively the rabbit should be given an analgesic injection. Analgesia should be continued for a few days if there is marked damage to the tongue or cheeks. If there is any tongue ulceration antibiotics should be given. As the teeth will regrow this may need to be repeated every 4–6 weeks; however, if the diet is improved to include more coarse fibre to promote chewing this interval may be lengthened. After the cheek teeth have been trimmed on several occasions, the damage to the crowns may be such that the teeth eventually stop growing leading to an apparent improvement in the condition.

Prevention: There has recently been a lot of interest in the part that diet, particularly dietary calcium, has to play in the aetiology of dental disease. The consistency of the diet is important. Plenty of fibre should be offered to promote chewing, and grass is even more abrasive than hay. The diet should not consist solely of a dry ration, which will cause the rabbit to chew with a crushing action, rather than a sideways action. Calcium is important, not only for tooth quality, but also for bone quality, and it is the latter that may predispose to malocclusion, as osteomalacia will lead to movement of the teeth within their sockets. The rabbit has an unusual calcium metabolism in that it absorbs calcium in direct proportion to the level of digestible calcium in the diet, and serum calcium rises in proportion to the absorbed calcium. The regulatory control via parathyroid hormone and vitamin D which is present in other species is absent in the rabbit. Any excess calcium is excreted in the urine, and if dietary calcium is high this may lead to calculi formation.

Pet rabbits on a mixed dry food, containing a mixture of cereals, peas, biscuits and pellets will often selectively pick out the cereals which are very low in calcium, and leave the pellets which contain the vitamins and minerals.

House rabbits or rabbits kept in sheds will not be able to synthesise their own vitamin D as they are not exposed to ultraviolet light. Vitamin D plays an essential part in the regulation of calcium uptake.

At present the best advice to prevent dental disease is as follows:

(1) To offer smaller quantities of dry food to ensure that all components are eaten, and that the rabbit does not selectively leave the pellets (which contain the calcium and vitamins).

(2) Selective feeders, or rabbits showing obvious calcification defects such as lines in the enamel of the upper incisors, can be given supplementation. A vitamin supplementation is best, as the vitamin D will enable dietary calcium to be absorbed. Vionate (Sherleys) or Arkvits (VetArk) can be used.

(3) Hay should be given as a good source of vitamin D, and to promote chewing.

(4) Greenstuff should be given daily; dandelions and clover are good sources of calcium.

(5) The rabbit should be allowed access to natural daylight every day.

THE MOUTH

Oral papilloma virus

This causes small, benign self-limiting tumours on the ventral surface of the tongue. These are spread by direct contact and oral trauma. These tumours are rare and generally regress after several weeks.

12 THE HEAD AND NECK

THE EYE

The rabbit has a 190° field of vision from each eye. This wide field of vision is possible as the eyes are sited on the top of the head. This position does mean that the rabbit is unable to see directly in front of its nose, and see what it is eating. Rabbits are also very long-sighted.

Some rabbits may sit and sway slowly back and forth, this may be referred to as 'scanning' or 'tracking'. By doing this the rabbit is causing motion in order to see an object close to itself, as head motion is thought to be a means of enhancing distance measurement.

Anatomy

The eye sits in a bony orbit. The tooth roots of the upper molars can impinge on this orbit and may cause retrobulbar abscesses. There is a large orbital venous sinus at the back of the orbit, and care must be taken to avoid this during surgery as it may bleed profusely.

Epiphora

Clinical signs: There is a clear watery discharge from both eyes. It may be the only symptom of atopy, or it may be associated with other clinical signs such as pruritis, crusting, and self-trauma of the ears, nose, feet, thighs and abdomen.

Chronic conjunctivitis and dacrocystitis can lead to scarring and blockage of the tear duct and subsequently persistent epiphora.

Dental disease can also cause epiphora if the incisor or first upper premolar roots press on the lacrimal duct.

Treatment: Dacrocystitis and dental disease must be identified and treated. Other cases of epiphora can be treated with steroid eye drops. If other signs of atopy are present parenteral corticosteroids can be given. The antihistamine diphenhydramine can be put in the drinking water (e.g. Benedryl elixir (Parke Davis & Co. Ltd.) at a dilution of 1:45 in the drinking water daily)

Prevention: Trigger factors should be eliminated. Any hay given should not be dusty. The hutch should be cleaned regularly to avoid the build-up of ammonia which is irritant to the eyes. A lower protein diet should be fed, as high protein diets are responsible for the formation of ammonia. Rabbits with persistent watery eyes benefit from a companion, as mutual grooming will keep the eyes clean.

Conjunctivitis

Clinical signs: Reddened conjunctiva, accompanied by a clear or purulent ocular discharge. There may be accompanying symptoms such as a tear duct infection, rhinitis or corneal ulceration. Trigger factors are those that cause epiphora.

A severe, purulent conjunctivitis is seen in cases of myxomatosis.

Treatment: The majority of cases of conjunctivitis are caused by *Staphylococcus aureus*. *Pasteurella* infections are also common. A topical eye preparation effective against *Staphylococcus* such as fusidic acid (Fucithalmic, Leo Laboratories Ltd.) should be used for 10–14 days. Longstanding cases of conjunctivitis may also require oral or parenteral antibiotics, preferably after bacterial culture.

If there is an accompanying tear duct infection the ducts should be flushed before antibiotic therapy.

Neonatal conjunctivitis

Clinical signs: One or more of a litter may be affected. The eyes are delayed in opening, and the eyelids are stuck together with a purulent discharge. The causal agent is usually *Staphylococcus aureus*. Subsequent litters from the same doe may be similarly affected.

Treatment: The eyelids should be gently bathed open with warm water. The cornea may be ulcerated. An antibiotic eye ointment such as fusidic acid (Fucithalmic, Leo Laboratories Ltd.) or chlortetracycline (Aureomycin ophthalmic ointment, Fort Dodge Animal Health) should be used until the condition resolves. Antibiotics may also be given orally or parenterally.

Dacrocystitis (tear duct infection)

Tear duct infections are common in rabbits. The nasolacrimal duct passes from the medial canthus of the eye over the roots of the first premolar and incisors to exit through the nares. Any tooth root abnormalities may lead to distortion and blockage of the tear duct, and secondary bacterial infection. Dacrocystitis may be one of the earliest indicators of dental disease. The bacteria most commonly isolated are *Staphylococcus* spp., *Streptococcus* spp. and *Pasteurella*, which can also be isolated from the nasal tracts of healthy rabbits.

Clinical signs: There is a thick white discharge from one or both eyes. If the lower eyelid is pulled out and pressure put on the medial canthus of the eye this discharge can be seen welling up from the lacrimal punctum. There may be an associated discharge from the corresponding nostril. There is generally a moderate to severe conjunctivitis, and some cases may not be able to open their eyelids. A secondary dermatitis may be present below the medial aspect of the eyes.

Treatment: Mild cases may respond to regular eye bathing, and the use of an antibiotic or antibiotic–corticosteroid eye preparation. A antibiotic effective against *Pasteurella* should be chosen. Gentamicin (Tiacil ophthalmic solution, Virbac Ltd.) is a good choice. The effectiveness of bathing will be increased if the discharge can be 'milked' from the duct by pressure on the medial canthus of the eye. The ventilation of the environment should be improved, and care should be taken not to allow ammonia to build up as this will be irritant to the eyes. An antibiotic such as enrofloxacin can be given orally for 7–10 days.

More severe cases will need flushing of the tear duct. If the infection is associated with obvious tooth root deformities, the rabbit may benefit from tooth extraction. A radiograph should help determine which tooth roots are responsible. A radiographic contrast medium can be flushed through the duct (one duct at a time) to determine the path of the duct.

Procedure for nasolacrimal duct flushing: This can be done under local anaesthetic alone, or with sedation and local anaesthetic. The lacrimal punctum is very obvious in the medial canthus of the eye, once the lower lid has been pulled down. Digital pressure below the punctum will help open the punctum and make it easier to place the catheter. The duct can be flushed with sterile saline. Flushing is successful when purulent material and then saline exit the nares. The purulent material can be collected on a sterile swab for bacterial culture and sensitivity if indicated. If the duct is very blocked the initial flushing may cause large amounts of purulent material to pour from the punctum. If the duct is disrupted the saline may leak into the surrounding tissues or go into the retrobulbar space causing the eye to bulge. If this occurs flushing should stop immediately. The saline should reabsorb over the next 24 hours, but the pressure behind the eye is initially painful and analgesia should be given.

Once successful flushing has been accomplished, an antibiotic–steroid eye preparation or diluted antibiotic solution can be placed in the duct via the canula, preferably an antibiotic effective against *Pasteurella*. After this procedure the rabbit is discharged with eye drops and antibiosis for 7–10 days. Gentamicin eye drops can be used twice daily, and are the drug of choice if a culture is not performed. Subsequent flushing may be necessary at daily or weekly intervals depending upon the severity of the condition.

If it not possible to flush the duct due to the presence of large quantities of purulent material a solution of trypsin can be instilled into the duct to attempt to break it down, and flushing can be reattempted after 48 hours. In practice, a solution of trypsin can be made by dissolving one capsule of pancreatic enzyme (e.g. Tryplase) in 5–10 ml of saline.

Corneal ulceration

Damage to the cornea is usually the result af abrasions from the hay or straw bedding. However, it is also a sequel of long-standing dacrocystitis. If the ulceration is severe it may result in desmatocoele formation and subsequent rupture of the globe.

Treatment: Most cases will respond to the use of a topical antibiotic eye preparation. Ulcers that do not respond to antibiotics may require debridement of any necrotic epithelium. The edges of the ulcer can be cauterised with phenol to stimulate healing. Severe cases may require enucleation.

Corneal lipidosis

Clinical signs: There are white fatty deposits on the cornea. These deposits can be anywhere on the cornea, and can vary in density. The lesions may be accompanied by corneal vascularisation.

Treatment: None required.

Corneal dystrophy

Clinical signs: Small grey opacities are seen on the centre of the cornea. They are caused by the thickening and disorganisation of the epithelial membrane.

Treatment: None required.

Keratitis

Rabbits can develop a severe keratitis, often secondary to dacrocystitis, or corneal trauma. The surface of the cornea may be almost completely covered with a white 'skin'. There is usually an accompanying conjunctivitis.

Treatment: This condition may respond to cephalexin given by sub-cutaneous injection at a dose of 20 mg/kg once daily for 5 days, and the use of a cephalonium containing eye ointment (Cepravin eye ointment, Schering-Plough Animal Health), used daily for up to 3 weeks.

Uveitis

Clinical signs: There are focal abscesses in the iris, or hypopyon and corneal oedema. This may be associated with *Pasteurella* infection, but can also be caused by other bacteria. Intraocular encephalitozoonosis has also been reported.

Treatment: A topical eye preparation containing chloramphenicol should be used. If the inflammation is diffuse antibiotics should also be given orally or parenterally. Topical corticosteroids may also be necessary to control the inflammation.

The prognosis for these cases is guarded. Enucleation should be considered if there is no response to treatment.

Entropion

This is caused by the inturning of the upper or lower eyelids, and is present from birth, although the symptoms may only become apparent at 2 weeks of age when the eyes open. The constant rubbing of the eyelashes on the cornea will lead to secondary corneal ulceration. Rex and Rex-cross rabbits are most prone to this condition.

Treatment: Any corneal ulceration should be managed with a topical antibiotic ointment until the rabbit is of a size that corrective surgery can be performed.

Harderian gland

Rabbits possess a Harderian gland which is situated behind the third eyelid. Rarely this gland may become inflamed or prolapse, so that there is a large red mass visible in the medial canthus of the eye. Antibiotic and anti-inflammatory treatment can be used topically, However if it does not respond to the treatment, or recurs regularly, then surgery should be considered. The area is very vascular and may bleed profusely during surgery.

Retrobulbar abscesses

These may be associated with tooth root infections, long-standing dacrocystitis, and the migration of foreign bodies such as hay seeds.

Clinical signs: Protrusion of the globe. The globe is of normal size, but is pushed outwards, in comparison with glaucoma where the globe itself is enlarged. There may be an associated rhinitis or dacrocystitis.

Treatment: Some cases will respond to aggressive antibiotic therapy, and in older patients long-term antibiosis may be the treatment of choice. Enucleation followed by flushing of the orbit is the alternative form of treatment.

Enucleation

Enucleation can be performed using the transconjunctival or transpalpebral approach. Care must be taken to avoid the venous sinus which will bleed profusely. If there is associated tooth root infection or osteomyelitis, the long-term prognosis must be guarded. Any infected tissue should be debrided once the globe has been removed. Post-operative antibiotics must be given orally or parenterally for 10–14 days.

   In circumstances where a second eye requires enucleation, rabbits have been seen to adjust extremely well, relying upon their senses of hearing, smell and touch.

Glaucoma

Glaucoma occurs as the intraocular pressure increases. Clinical signs are often unilateral initially; however, often both eyes are affected. The affected eye looks swollen, the pupillary light response becomes delayed, and as the condition advances corneal oedema develops.

Glaucoma is hereditary in New Zealand White rabbits and the symptoms can occur as early as 3–5 months of age.

Treatment: Trusopt drops 1% (Merck, Sharp and Dohme Ltd.), which contain 22.3 mg/ml dorzolamide hydrochloride, can be used in the eye at a rate of one drop every 24 hours. Dichlorphenamide can also be given at a dose of 1–2 mg/kg daily. If the response to these drugs is poor, then enucleation is recommended. Affected rabbits should not be bred from.

Cataracts

A cataract is an opacity of the lens. Some cataracts are congenital, and some develop later in life. Cataracts can be unilateral or bilateral. Surgery is unnecessary in the pet rabbit as it can cope adequately with poor vision.

THE EAR

The ears of wild rabbits are their most important sensory organ. Both ears can move independently, and their large surface area can funnel sound waves into the ear; even sounds of very low volume can be detected. Evolution and selective breeding mean that the ears of pet rabbits are diverse, from the short prick ears of the Netherland Dwarf to the English Lop whose ear span can be as much as 70 cm; consequently their effectiveness for receiving sound waves may be diminished in certain breeds. Normal rabbit ear wax is golden and non-odorous; any variation indicates a disease process, the commonest of which is infection with *Psoroptes cuniculi*.

Ear mites

Clinical signs: Early cases may have mildly pruritic ears, and rabbits can carry low grade infections for long periods of time. More advanced cases have thick yellow–grey crusts in the ears, which are very inflamed. The condition is pruritic. Rarely the lesions may spread across the face and limbs. Crusty lesions have also been reported on the ventral abdomen around the vent. In this site it must be differentiated from treponemiasis (rabbit syphilis).

Diagnosis: Microscopy. The mite will be present in large numbers in the lesions. They may be visible to the naked eye as they may reach 0.7 mm in size. Examination under the microscope reveals their oval body shape, pointed mouthparts and three jointed pedicles with funnel shaped suckers.

Treatment: Ivermectin is given by subcutaneous injection at a dose of 400 μg/kg. The injection should be repeated on two more occasions at fortnightly intervals, as the mite takes 21 days to complete its life cycle. If the ears are to be cleaned, the rabbit should be sedated as removal of the crusts is very painful. The ears and skin can be bathed with dilute chlorhexidine, although there is no actual need to do this as once treatment has begun the crusts will dry up and fall out after a few days. A short-acting corticosteroid can be given by injection to limit the inflammation. A few drops of 1% ivermectin can also be put directly into each ear.

   In-contact rabbits should also be treated, and the environment must be disinfected and sprayed with an acaricide, as the female mites can live off the host for several weeks making reinfestation possible.

Otitis

Clinical signs: There is a white viscous exudate, often from one ear only.

Treatment: Antibiotics may be given orally, preferably based on the results of a culture test. Aural preparations can be used, and the ear can be flushed with a dilute chlorhexidine solution.

Warts

These are common on the pinna. They are benign and no treatment is necessary.

THE NECK

Head tilt ('wry neck')

Rabbits are commonly presented with a sudden onset head tilt (torticollis). There are several possible causes for this condition, which may be difficult to differentiate in the live rabbit; a full diagnosis is often only possible at post-mortem. Cases associated with inner ear infection or cerebrovascular accidents may improve over several months, and the rabbit may learn to compensate for the head tilt. One complication is that the down-side eye may develop corneal ulceration as it rubs on the floor, and this will require appropriate treatment. Rabbits with a head tilt should be handled as little as possible, as when they are picked up they lose all spatial awareness and may begin to spin. Once their feet are replaced to the floor they can regain their balance. If it is necessary to pick them up they should be held as close to the body as possible.

Causes of head tilt

Infection: Otitis media and otitis interna are generally caused by *Pasteurella* infection, but *Staphylococcus*, *Pseudomonas*, *Bordetella bronchiseptica*, *Bacteroides* and *Escherichia coli* have been isolated from ear infections.

Pus may be evident in the ear canal, and on radiography the tympanic bullae which are normally thin-walled and hollow develop an increased soft tissue opacity and thicker walls. Otitis interna may be accompanied by horizontal nystagmus (compared with central vestibular disease which is accompanied by vertical nystagmus).

Treatment with long-term antibiotics is necessary. Most infections are sensitive to enrofloxacin, and this can be given orally. It may take 4–6 weeks before an improvement is seen, and antibiotics may need to be given for 6 months or longer.

A bulla osteotomy can be performed if there is a large amount of purulent material in the middle ear to allow permanent drainage from the bulla.

Cerebrovascular accident *(stroke):* This is the second most common cause of head tilt, after otitis. The onset is sudden, and the rabbit may move in circles. Nystagmus is present in some cases.

A short-acting corticosteroid can be given. Long-term use of corticosteroids is contraindicated as this may trigger latent *Pasteurella* infection. Antibiotics should be given to rule out infection.

These rabbits need intensive nursing, but may improve over time. Many compensate for the head tilt, and are able to eat and drink with some support.

Encephalitozoonosis: Encephalitozoonosis is caused by the protozoal parasite *Encephalitozoon cuniculi*. Spores have a predilection for kidney and brain tissue. Neurological symptoms include head tilt, tremors, posterior paresis, convulsions and death. (See separate section below.)

Trauma: Any injury to the head can lead to brain injury. If the trauma is not too severe a short-acting corticosteroid injection can be given to reduce any inflammation.

Neoplasia: Neoplasia of the brain, neck or ear is not commonly recorded, but a lesion in one of these sites will cause a head tilt.

Toxicity: Lead poisoning can cause a head tilt. House rabbits may have access to sources of lead (e.g. paints, curtain weights) and lead poisoning should be considered as a differential diagnosis in these cases. Occasionally lead can be seen on abdominal radiographs if it has recently been ingested. (See Chapter 13.)

Cerebral nematodiasis: Cerebral larvae migrans can be caused by *Baylisascaris procyonis*, the common roundworm of the raccoon and skunk. The eggs can remain infective for up to 1 year, and the common source for rabbits is contaminated hay and greenfoods. The eggs are ingested by the rabbit and migrating larvae enter the brain tissue, and cause destruction of the nervous tissue. Neurological signs include head tilt, ataxia, circling and tremors. Anisocoria (uneven pupils) is another symptom of central nervous system involvement. There is no effective treatment for this condition. Ivermectin can be given; it may kill the migrating larvae, but is unlikely to penetrate the brain to reach the larvae in the brain tissue. In areas where the racoon is prevalent it is important to prevent faecal contamination of food and hay by the raccoon.

Encephalitozoonosis

Encephalitozoonosis is caused by the protozoal parasite *Encephalitozoon cuniculi*. The disease is sometimes referred to as nosematosis, as the organism was previously named *Nosema cuniculi*. The majority of infections are subclinical, and many rabbits are seropositive for the disease without showing any clinical signs. The development of the disease depends upon the infective dose, and the host resistance. Young rabbits of 4–6 weeks are most vulnerable. Dwarf rabbits are more susceptible than larger breeds.

Encephalitozoonosis is considered a zoonotic risk for humans that are already immunosuppressed.

Life-cycle: The life cycle is 3–5 weeks, and antibodies are only made once the life cycle is complete. Spores are shed in the urine for 2–3 months post-infection. The spores are transmitted by ingestion or inhalation. It is possible there is also some transplacental spread. The spores have a predilection for kidney and brain tissue; however, they may spread to other organs such as the liver and lungs. Infective spores appear in the urine 35 days after infection.

Clinical signs: The majority of infections are subclinical, but when the infective dose is high the symptoms reflect the sites in which the spores are found. Neurological signs caused by the granulomatous lesions are most common and include head tilt, posterior paresis, paralysis, tremors, ataxia and convulsions. Less commonly, signs of kidney infection may be seen as polydipsia, polyuria and weight loss.

Once antibodies are produced the organism is killed, but the clinical signs reflect the tissue damage that is caused as the protozoan multiplies.

Diagnosis: Diagnosis is made by the demonstration of spores by histopathology, or by detection of antibodies by ELISA or IFA tests. The interpretation of antibody tests is difficult due to the presence of healthy seropositive rabbits. The detection of antibodies does not always mean that *E. cuniculi* is the cause of the disease; however, a zero titre would rule it out of a differential diagnosis. A rising titre would indicate recent infection; antibodies first appear 4 weeks post-infection, and peak at 9 weeks.

Treatment: There is no treatment other than supportive care. Recently metronidazole has been tried, and albendazole. The dose of albendazole is 15 mg/kg orally once a day. This is not licensed for rabbits and the effects of long term use are not known.

The use of tetracyclines may suppress the protozoan, but do not eliminate it. Tetracyclines can be given via the drinking water at a dose of 500 mg/litre, or orally at a dose rate of 20 mg/kg twice daily.

Mild clinical cases may respond to a high dose of steroids, e.g. 2 mg/kg of dexamethasone.

Prevention: The spores survive for 6 weeks at 22°C (71°F), but for less than 1 week at 4°C (39°F). They can survive for a month in dry conditions. As they are spread in the urine, good sanitation is extremely important, especially when a doe has young kits that are most vulnerable. Disinfection of the hutches with a quaternary ammonium solution or 0.3% bleach should inactivate the spores.

Urinary contamination of food and water can be avoided by using hay racks and sipper bottles, and by raising the food dishes from the floor.

THE DEWLAP

The dewlap is a large fold of skin over the throat. Although it is normal, it is often presented as a concern by owners. It is seen in older female rabbits, and can become extremely large, particularly in obese animals. Breeding females, and those exhibiting pseudopregnancy, will pluck fur from this area to line their nest.

Moist dermatitis often develops in this area (see Chapter 4). This is often associated with chronic moistening of the dewlap and infection with *Pseudomonas aeruginosa* ('blue fur disease').

Lumps may appear in the dewlap. Around 90% of these are normal fatty deposits. Abscesses can occur; these can be identified by the aspiration of purulent material, and are best treated by complete surgical excision and antibiotics.

Cellulitis will present as a painful oedematous swelling of the neck accompanied by pyrexia (40–42°C; 104–108°F). As the condition progresses the skin may become necrotic. This should be treated with aggressive antibiosis and analgesia. Cool baths will help relieve the discomfort.

Neoplasia is rare.

Dewlap reduction

Occasionally the dewlap can become so large that it can hinder normal physiological processes. The rabbit may be unable to practice caecotrophy, resulting in 'sticky bottom syndrome'. The rabbit may also be unable to groom itself; when bringing its forepaws up to its face it may become smothered by this flap of skin, and ineffectually rub hair from the dewlap in its attempt to wash itself. The rabbit may pluck hair from this area in frustration. These cases are candidates for dewlap reduction.

The rabbit is anaethetised and placed in dorsal recumbency and prepared for surgery. A large elliptical incision is made at right angles to the midline, ending medially to the point of each shoulder. The large flap of skin is removed, and skin closure is routine. The author closes the skin in three or four sections with a continuous apposition suture which is accepted better by the rabbit than simple interrupted sutures.

13 NEUROLOGICAL AND NEUROMUSCULAR DISORDERS

Clinical signs of neuromuscular disorders include depression, torticollis, paresis and paralysis. Each symptom separately can be attributed to many different disease conditions, which may be covered in greater detail elsewhere in the text. This section aims to provide a comprehensive list of differential diagnoses for each symptom.

DEPRESSION

This generally occurs secondary to a non-neurological problem. Any depressed rabbit carries a poor prognosis, as it can lose the will to live. The underlying cause must be investigated; analgesia is important as often low-grade pain is the cause of anorexia and depression. Fluids must be given, and the rabbit force fed if necessary. Companionship in the form of another rabbit, particularly if the rabbit is pair-bonded, is essential.

TORTICOLLIS

The possible causes of torticollis ('wry neck' or 'head tilt') are otitis media/interna, cerebrovascular accidents, trauma, neoplasia, encephalitozoonosis, toxoplasmosis, or intoxication (see Chapter 12).

Otitis media/interna

This is the most common cause of torticollis. If the tympanic membrane has ruptured pus will be evident in the ear canal. Diagnosis may require radiography of the tympanic bullae, and culture of the pus. The most common causal agents are *Pasteurella multocida* and *Staphylococcus* spp. Treatment requires long-term antibiotics.

Cerebrovascular accidents ('stroke')

This will result in a head tilt, horizontal nystagmus, weakness of one side and circling. A single dose of corticosteroids can be given initially, and the patient will require careful nursing. The condition may gradually improve over time.

Encephalitozoonosis

This is caused by the protozoan *Encephalitozoon cuniculi*. A non-suppurative meningitis can occur; the initial symptoms are torticollis and tremors, which progress to a chronic progressive paralysis, convulsions and coma. The organism has a predilection for renal and brain tissue, and renal and central nervous system disease may occur concurrently. Renal symptoms include polydipsia, polyuria, a loss of litter training, incontinence and urine scald.

Neoplasia

Neoplasia of the central nervous system includes medullary and pituitary teratomas and pituitary adenomas. Central brain lesions are often accompanied by vertical nystagmus.

Cerebral nematodiasis

In areas where the raccoon is a wild animal, cerebral nematodiasis is possible. This is caused by larvae from *Baylisascaris procyonis*, the common roundworm of raccoons. The rabbit becomes infected via food or bedding contaminated by raccoon faeces. The larvae migrans are found in the cerebellum, cerebrum, mid-brain and medulla; symptoms include torticollis, circling, ataxia, opisthotonos and tremors. The contamination of food and bedding by raccoons must be prevented, as the eggs of *B. procyonis* are capable of surviving for a year in the environment.

Listeriosis

Listeriosis, caused by the bacterium *Listeria monocytogenes* is rare, but has been reported. The organism causes a brain stem meningoencephalitis and causes rolling and torticollis.

PARESIS AND PARALYSIS

Spinal trauma

The most common cause of paresis is spinal trauma. Vertebral fractures can occur through improper handling, as the rabbit twists its spine. Caged rabbits with osteoporosis associated with limited exercise can suffer a vertebral fracture through foot stamping when frightened or startled. The commonest site for fractures is L6 and L7. Other vertebral disorders include vertebral luxations, osteomyelitis, discospondylitis, arthritis and spondylosis.

Clinical signs of vertebral disorders are paresis, paraplegia, urinary incontinence or retention. There may be loss of motor and sensory response to the limbs, and loss of anal sphincter tone. The diagnosis should be confirmed by radiography. The decision to treat or euthanase should be based on the degree of spinal cord damage. Rabbits that retain some motor function may respond to corticosteroid and diuretic therapy.

'Splay leg'

'Splay leg' is a term that is used to describe any condition that results in the failure to adduct one or more legs. The hind legs are most commonly affected, and may be only capable of weak uncoordinated movements, or be completely paralysed. The cause of splay leg is developmental, and the condition is seen in young rabbits up to a few months of age. Possible developmental abnormalities include hypoplasia pelvis, femoral luxation or subluxation, hip and shoulder achondroplasia and distal foreleg curvature. If more than one leg is affected, euthanasia is the kindest option. If a single leg is affected in a pet rabbit, the rabbit may well be able to cope with its disability, and amputation of the limb can be considered when the rabbit is old enough to withstand a general anaesthetic.

Toxoplasmosis

Toxoplasmosis caused by infection by *Toxoplasma gondii* is a rare cause of posterior paralysis. Other symptoms include ataxia and muscle tremors. The paralysis may progress to paraplegia. The neurological symptoms are associated with bradyzoites in the central nervous system. In older rabbits cysts in the central nervous system are associated with a granulomatous encephalitis.

Infection is via food and bedding contaminated with cat faeces; also from soil and unwashed vegetables. Cats should be kept from soiling the rabbit's environment at all times.

METABOLIC DISORDERS

Hypercalcaemia

Hypercalcaemia has been seen in some rabbits with paresis, and these rabbits may respond to a low calcium diet, or diuresis. The actual significance of the hypercalcaemia is unknown.

Hypokalaemia

A flaccid paresis can be due to hypokalaemia. Normal blood potassium levels are 3.6–6.9 mg/dl. These rabbits can respond dramatically to the oral administration of tomato juice. They can be given up to 10 ml three times daily.

INHERITED DISORDERS

Inherited disorders are rare, but can result in a range of neurological disorders. Shaking palsy results in tremor and flaccid paralysis, and paralytic tremor results in progressive spastic paralysis. 'Waltzing' is a disorder which causes the rabbit to circle.

OTHER DISORDERS WITH NEUROLOGICAL SIGNS

Hydrocephalus

This can be an inherited disorder, it can also occur in hypo- and hypervitaminosis A. The affected rabbit may show circling, convulsions, opisthotonos and paralysis.

Lead poisoning

This is now more common since more rabbits are kept free range indoors with potential access to lead in old paint, curtain weights, the foil around wine bottles, etc.

Clinical signs: These may be vague and include anorexia, lethargy and neurological changes. Anorexia and weight loss are the most common symptoms.

Diagnosis: An abdominal radiograph may show ingested metal in the abdomen. A blood sample for lead levels should be taken, and haematology may reveal basophilic stippling of the red blood cells.

Treatment: Rabbits with a blood lead level greater than 10 µg/dl should be treated with injections of calcium versenate (Ca-EDTA). The dose is 27.5 mg/kg by subcutaneous injection four times a day for 5 days. A second course may be required a week later.

Heat stroke

Rabbits are particularly susceptible to heat stroke, and this is an important factor to consider when planning their environment. They should not be exposed to direct sunlight in the heat of the day without some shade and shelter being provided. Indoor cages should not be placed directly by a radiator or window.

Clinical signs: Respiratory distress, mouth breathing, weakness, depression, incoordination and convulsions. Body temperature more than 40.5°C (105°F).

Treatment: The rabbit should be sprayed with a water spray or immersed in tepid water. Fluids should be given by intravenous or subcutaneous injection. A shock dose of dexamethasone (2 mg/kg) can be given intravenously.

Pregnancy toxaemia (ketosis)

This is a rare condition, seen in overweight does in their last week of pregnancy.

Clinical signs: Lethargy, dullness of the eyes, salivation, respiratory distress, convulsions and collapse. The breath may have the classic acetone smell of ketosis. The urine becomes acidic (pH 5–6).

Treatment: Glucose should be given orally, or as a subcutaneous or intraperitoneal injection of 5% glucose. A short-acting corticosteroid injection may be beneficial. The rabbit can be force fed baby cereal and fruit purée.

Rabies

Rabbits are capable of contracting rabies, but actual cases are rare. It should be considered in any area where rabies may be endemic in the wild fox or skunk population. Clinical signs are neurological and include blindness and forelimb paralysis. Pet rabbits must be protected from wild animals in areas where rabies is endemic.

Epilepsy

True epilepsy is rare in rabbits; however, seizures can occur secondary to other disease processes. Encephalitis associated with *Pasteurella* infection can result in seizures. Ketosis, resulting from hepatic lipidosis can cause convulsions, as can azotemia associated with renal dysfunction.

14   IMPORTANT VIRAL DISEASES

RABBIT HAEMORRHAGIC VIRUS DISEASE (HVD)

Historical background

HVD was first identified in China in 1984, and has since spread across Europe, with the first case being reported in Britain in 1992. It was made a notifiable disease by the *Special Diseases (Notification) Order* in 1991, but regulations were later removed in October 1996. The first British case of HVD in a wild rabbit was reported in October 1994, and it is now thought to be endemic in the wild rabbit population in both mainland Europe and Great Britain.

The virus

HVD is caused by a calicivirus. The virus replicates within the hepatocytes of the liver causing hepatic necrosis. The damaged hepatocytes release tissue thromboplastins which initiate disseminated intravascular coagulation, which is responsible for the haemorrhages seen in other organs, notably the lungs and kidneys. The subsequent intracapillary micro-thrombosis, particularly of the lungs, leads to the development of the clinical symptoms.

Transmission

The virus is present in the saliva and nasal secretions of affected rabbits. It can be spread by direct and indirect contact. Mechanical transmission may be via insects, birds, rodents, people and their clothing, and contaminated feed and water equipment. Studies have shown that the virus can survive for at least 3 months on clothing. The spread from Europe to Britain may have been via birds, aerosol transmission, or considering the proximity of the first outbreaks to the coast, by cross-channel ferry traffic.

Clinical signs

Only rabbits over 6 weeks of age are affected. This may be due to the resistant nature of the hepatocytes in the neonate, or the presence of maternal immunity at this time. Rabbits between 4 and 6 weeks may show transient symptoms but will survive. In older rabbits the morbidity may be as high as 30–60%, and the mortality of affected animals may reach 100%. The incubation period is 16 hours–3 days. There are three different clinical presentations.

Peracute: Sudden death 1–2 days post-infection. Death may precede the clinical signs, or the rabbit may die convulsing with epistaxis.

Acute: Anorexia, lethargy, dyspnoea 2–3 days post-infection. The rabbit will die convulsing with epistaxis. Some rabbits may scream with pain.

Mild: This occurs with transient infection. The rabbit is lethargic and partially anorexic. Recovery is spontaneous, and these rabbits are resistant to re-infection. These rabbits may develop secondary infections such as diarrhoea, or 'snuffles'.

   Antibodies are passed in the colostrum and are transferred to suckling rabbits.

Diagnosis

Diagnosis can be confirmed by virus isolation. Post-mortem changes may be highly suggestive of the disease. The liver will be swollen, friable and a brownish-red colour. There may be haemorrhages on the liver, kidneys, spleen, heart and lymph nodes. Petechial haemorrhages will be found over the surface of the lungs, which may be covered in a blood-tinged foamy exudate. There may be blood from the nostrils, and haemorrhages and bloody fluid in the trachea.

Treatment

None is possible for the per-acute and acute stages of the disease. Mild cases need supportive treatment and treatment of any secondary infections.

Control

Vaccination: This is the best control measure. The vaccine available is an oil adjuvanated vaccine containing inactivated HVD virus. Rabbits can be vaccinated from 10–12 weeks of age and given annual booster injections. The skin should be massaged at the injection site after vaccination to prevent a skin reaction developing. Rabbits kept outside appear to be at most risk from the virus, but even house rabbits should be vaccinated as they can still be exposed to passive carriers.

Hygiene: Cages should be cleaned regularly. Antec Virkon (Alstoe Animal Health) contains 50% potassium peroxomonosulphate, 5% sulphamic acid and 15% sodium alkyl benzene sulphonate; it claims to be effective against calicivirus. Unfortunately other effective disinfectants are 10% formalin, or 1% sodium hydroxide, both of which are toxic to the operator. The virus can withstand 50°C (122°F) for at least 6 minutes.

Elimination of passive carriers: Insects, birds, rodents and other animals should be kept away from the rabbit's environment.

Avoidance of contaminated foodstuffs: Do not pick greenfoods from areas frequented by wild rabbits.

MXYOMATOSIS

Historical background

Myxomatosis is endemic in South American rabbits. It was deliberately introduced from Brazil to Australia in the 1950s where it caused a devastating epidemic and is now endemic. The disease gradually spread across Europe to Great Britain where it is now endemic in the wild population, and can cause up to 100% mortality if it infects pet rabbits.

The virus

The myxoma virus is a pox virus. The virus is introduced into the skin of the rabbit by a biting insect. The virus moves to a local lymph node, and then to several skin sites via the bloodstream. The virus multiplies in the skin around the eyes, nose, base of the ears and the genitals.

Transmission

The disease is spread by blood sucking insects. In Great Britain the main vector is the rabbit flea, whilst in other countries the mosquito is the major vector. Although rabbits kept outside are at the most risk, house rabbits are also vulnerable because other domestic pets, especially cats, can carry the fleas indoors. Myxomatosis does not appear to be spread by simple contact of two rabbits, but it relies on the carriage by an insect vector between the rabbits. The virus can remain alive in the blood of fleas for many months, and hence the disease can persist from year to year as the fleas overwinter in rabbit burrows, or in the rabbit's home environment.

Clinical signs

The incubation period is 5–14 days. There are two presentations of the disease.

Acute form: The rabbit develops oedematous swellings around the eyes, base of the ears and genitals. The swelling of the genitals is pathognomic for myxomatosis. There is a purulent blepharo-conjunctivitis which progresses to blindness. The rabbit may maintain its appetite initially, but will become anorexic as the disease progresses. Secondary *Pasteurella* pneumonia is very common and the usual cause of death.

Chronic (nodular) form: The rabbit develops oedematous swellings (pseudo-tumours), especially on the ears, nose and paws, 10–15 days after infection. These will spontaneously resolve, although the resultant scabs take longer to disappear.

Diagnosis

The genital swelling is pathognomic for the disease, and the clinical signs of both forms are so typical that further diagnosis is not necessary. Virus isolation can be performed.

Treatment

The acute form of the disease can cause 100% mortality, and affected individuals are best euthanased. Treatment of less severe cases can be tried; intensive nursing is required, and long-term antibiotics to combat the secondary pneumonia. Affected animals may take weeks or months to recover, and the resultant scabs and scars may remain long after recovery.

The chronic form is self-limiting, and affected rabbits generally recover. Antibiosis may be necessary to limit any secondary infection.

Control

The disease can be controlled by two methods.

Vaccination: A vaccine is available that contains live Shope fibroma virus, which is closely related to the myxoma virus, but does not cause disease. At least part of the vaccine should be given intradermally for maximum effect. Rabbits can be injected from 6 weeks of age, and boosters should be given annually. In areas where myxomatosis is rife, vaccination can be repeated every 6 months. It is important to vaccinate both indoor and outdoor rabbits.

Insect control: Flea control is important, not only of the rabbit, but in the case of the house rabbit by treatment of other in-contact pets and the environment.

Mosquitos must also be controlled, by the use of mosquito netting in shed doors, and by the use of insect repellent strips. Rabbits kept outdoors should not have their runs placed in damp areas or near water sources, as these are areas of dense mosquito population.

Atypical myxomatosis

Rabbits that have partial immunity, or vaccinated rabbits in the face of overwhelming challenge may develop an atypical form of mxyomatosis. The rabbit develops cutaneous nodules in the absence of the more classic oedema of the eyelids and genital region. These rabbits may respond to nursing and antibiotics to prevent secondary *Pasteurella* infection. The nodules will develop a scab, and begin to heal, although the whole process may take as long as 10 weeks.

15 BEHAVIOUR

INTRODUCTION

Rabbits are becoming more popular as pets, and particularly if they are kept indoors we are more able to observe their behaviour. Although pet rabbits may seem to have evolved and changed in appearance from their wild ancestors their behaviour is still remarkably similar, and often the reasons for certain behaviour patterns can be explained with an understanding of the behaviour of their wild counterparts.

This chapter aims to discuss the most common behaviour problems, and normal behaviour patterns that may be perceived as a problem. There is now an Association of Pet Behaviour Counsellors, whose members are trained to give advice on problem behaviour, and the number of rabbit referrals for behaviour is increasing, as owners seek to solve problems, rather than opt to rehome a 'problem rabbit'.

Rabbits are natural prey animals, and in the wild they are constantly alert and ready to react to being caught by a predator. When they are scared they have three behaviour options, the fright, flight or fight response. In certain situations they may exhibit these responses which, if they become exaggerated, may become labelled as problem behaviour. In any situation it is important to look at it from the rabbit's point of view, and often its response can be explained by the natural behaviour of its wild ancestors.

Due to the placement of their eyes, rabbits cannot see well in front of their nose. It is this reason that they should not be offered a hand to sniff as we would to a dog, as they are more likely to nip the hand mistaking it for food.

BEHAVIOUR CHANGES AT SEXUAL MATURITY

The onset of sexual maturity can trigger many behavioural changes, the majority of which will be considered 'problem' behaviour by the owner.

Does reach sexual maturity when they are on average 80% of their adult body weight. This may be 3–4 months for the dwarf breeds and 5–7 months for the larger breeds. The doe may become aggressive, have mood swings, mount or fight its companions, spray like a buck, or begin digging and nesting.

The buck becomes sexually mature between 4 and 5 months of age, and may show mounting, spraying and aggression. Both sexes may lose their house trained habits.

Neutering is important to prevent this behaviour, ideally before the problem arises. Rabbits can be neutered before or as soon as they reach sexual maturity. Bucks can be castrated as soon as the testicles descend at around 14 weeks, and does can be spayed from 20 weeks.

Neutering should also help older rabbits that already exhibit undesirable behaviour. The loss of negative sexual behaviour is not immediate; many will improve within 2 weeks of surgery; for some rabbits, often the larger breeds, it may take up to 6 months. However, if the undesirable behaviour is sexual in origin, neutering will help. If the rabbit continues to be aggressive, other causes of aggression must be considered, such as fear or pain.

COMMON BEHAVIOUR PROBLEMS

Territory marking

Rabbits can mark their territory in three ways. Their hard droppings are coated in anal gland secretions, and left at several sites in their environment. The size of the environment determines how many sites are chosen. A rabbit in a small hutch may only use one site, whereas a rabbit allowed free run of a house may chose several sites. It is this feature that makes rabbits easy to litter train. If a rabbit passes droppings in places other than the litter tray it may be because the environment is large, and there are an insufficient number of trays. Adolescent rabbits may scatter droppings everywhere as they reach sexual maturity, and these rabbits will improve following neutering. Neutered rabbits are easiest to litter train, as they have less of an urge to mark multiple sites, and at this stage may be content to use just one or two trays.

Rabbits may also spray their territory, although this is an infrequent problem when compared with cats. Bucks, and occasionally does will spray, and neutering will correct this behaviour. Spraying is more commonly a sign of affection (see below).

Rabbits also have active scent glands under their chin, and will mark familiar and new objects by rubbing their chin on the object, known as 'chinning'. This is harmless behaviour, and is practised by both neutered and un-neutered rabbits. Occasionally the chin may become matted with the grease, and require gentle cleaning.

Spraying

Infrequently rabbits may spray to mark their territory. More commonly they spray objects for which they feel affection. This is almost exclusively a behavioural characteristic of the buck. The rabbit may spray its companion rabbit, or guinea pig, or may spray its owner. The rabbit may circle around the object of its affection and spray on the move with a flick of its hind-quarters. Rabbits may also spray on a submissive companion. Neutering before sexual maturity will prevent this problem. If spraying behaviour is already established in an adult male, neutering should cure the problem, although it may take up to 6 months for the behaviour to stop.

Response to handling

Most rabbits do not like to be picked up, although they are generally very affectionate once sitting on a lap, or beside their owner. This is because the only time a wild rabbit is picked up, it is by a predator who is going to eat it. The rabbit is genuinely scared and may exhibit one of three behaviour patterns.

(1) *Fright*. The rabbit crouches flat to the ground, cringing. This rabbit can be picked up with one hand on the scruff, and one hand supporting its bottom whilst reassuring it with a quiet voice.
(2) *Flight*. The rabbit runs away, and in the ensuing chase becomes even more frightened.
(3) *Fight*. The rabbit stands its ground and exhibits fear aggression.

These fears may be compounded by other factors. If the rabbit is only used to female hands and voices, it will be scared if handled by a man. Rabbits are also sensitive to certain smells, and are frightened by heavy perfumes, and the smell of oil and diesel.

Solutions

Once a rabbit is frightened of being picked up it may take a lot of time and effort to gain its trust. First the rabbit should become used to being close to and stroked by its owner before an attempt is made to pick it up. This may mean the owner sitting quietly on the floor with it, relying on its natural inquisitive nature which will lead it to sniff and explore its owner, and at this stage it can be enticed onto the lap with some treats.

The rabbit should also become used to being stroked, initially without any attempt to pick it up. Rabbits may be scared of hands approaching from in front of their faces, and the hand should approach from directly on top of the head, so that the rabbit feels rather than sees the hand. When two rabbits groom each other they groom the top of the head, the top of the nose, the ears, and down the back. Stroking in these areas is most likely to be interpreted by the rabbit as a friendly gesture rather than a threat.

If the rabbit exhibits fear aggression so that it bites the hand that approaches it, then stroking can be achieved with a long handled brush. The rabbit should be rewarded with food treats at the same time. Gradually the handle can be shortened, until the owner can stroke the rabbit.

Once the rabbit accepts stroking, it can be taught to be picked up. Initially it can be held supported with both hands and lifted just off the ground, and then put down again and rewarded. This process can be gradually built on until the rabbit can be picked up without struggling.

Whilst a rabbit is learning to trust its owner, confrontation should be avoided. If necessary ramps can be built to allow the rabbit to move from its hutch to exercise area avoiding the need to be picked up.

Prevention

It is very important that in the early socialisation phase around weaning that a rabbit is regularly handled. Handling should be done by both sexes so that the rabbit does not become frightened later.

Aggression

One of the commonest reasons that rabbits are taken to rabbit sanctuaries for rehoming is because they have become aggressive. If the reason for the aggression can be determined then the behaviour can usually be modified.

Territorial aggression

Rabbits that attack their owners when they are in their hutch are thought to display territorial aggression. This may occur seasonally, such as seen with entire does as they reach sexual maturity and during the breeding season, or as the result of pseudopregnancy. For these does neutering will calm their behaviour.

Rabbits that attack hands that approach them as they sit in their hutch may actually be exhibiting fear aggression towards the hand, rather than territorial aggression. As discussed in the section on handling, rabbits are fearful of hands that approach from their sides or face, and of hands that smell unusual. The hand should always approach from above or behind the head, and often the living quarters can be adapted to incorporate a top opening door to make this possible.

Food aggression

Rabbits may defend their food bowl, and attack the hand that tries to remove it. In the wild the rabbit is accustomed to a poor diet, and if it finds an area of lush grass it is its instinct to protect it. Rabbits that guard one food bowl in the same manner should be given many sources of food around their environment, so that one single site does not become so important. Fresh food can be scattered around, allowing the rabbit to develop its natural instinct to forage for food. Rabbits that are provided with a natural high fibre diet of hay and leafy vegetables that takes them several hours to forage for and graze on are likely to be more satisfied that the rabbit that receives its daily ration as a bowl of concentrated food which it can eat in less than half an hour. Diets that are rich in protein and carbohydrate (concentrate ration) are in themselves likely to cause behaviour problems. This is equivalent to feeding enough protein and carbohydrate to a racehorse, and then expecting it to be content to stand in a stable all day.

Fear aggression

The rabbit is a prey animal, and is naturally fearful of predators, and in particular of being chased, caught and picked up (see response to handling). When a rabbit is scared it can let out a high pitched scream. In the wild this scream is thought to warn other members of the colony, whilst attempting to frighten the predator.

In any situation that a rabbit may show aggression it is important to analyse the events to determine if the aggression is a fear response, and only then can the behaviour be modified by removal of the fearful stimulus.

Rabbits rely heavily on their hearing to give them early warning signals from the environment. Deafness is a common cause of fear, and fear aggression. This may be due to an inner ear infection, or more commonly a heavy build up of wax and pain associated with an ear mite infection. The ears should be examined and treated as necessary.

Sexual aggression

A rabbit can become aggressive once it reaches sexual maturity. This aggression may be towards other companions, or towards its owner. In does this aggression may be cyclical, relating to nest building and pseudopregnancy. Does with litters may show aggression when protecting their young, or a doe may protect other submissive companions. Does that may have uterine hyperplasia or adenocarcinoma can become aggressive. Aggression related to sexual maturity will greatly improve after neutering.

Pain aggression

Rabbits that are in pain will become short-tempered and aggressive. This pain may be from any source, and must be investigated accordingly.

COMMUNICATION

Nipping

Rabbits may nip to communicate with other rabbits, or if a house rabbit, to communicate with the other animals and humans that it lives with. It can also be used as an attention-seeking device. Rabbits also groom each other quite determinedly, and if this behaviour is redirected to a human companion it may result in a misdirected bite. If such a nip is painful the best response may be a piercing scream, to mimic natural rabbit communication, and teach the rabbit that this behaviour is undesirable.

Licking

Licking is another form of communication. It is mistakenly thought that rabbits lick because they are deficient in salt. However, licking is a variant of grooming behaviour and is a sign of affection.

Thumping

Thumping or stamping the hind legs is the way rabbits communicate fear to each other. In the wild when several rabbits are out grazing they will be alert for signs of danger. A thump of the feet will send all the rabbits back to the burrow. Similarly pet rabbits will stamp their feet if they sense danger. For rabbits that are on a healthy diet and allowed plenty of free exercise this activity poses no problems; however, for hutch rabbits thumping can be potentially dangerous. These rabbits may be suffering from osteoporosis and can sustain vertebral fractures and hind-limb paralysis through stamping.

This natural method of communication can be employed by the owner to their rabbit when the rabbit has free run of the house or garden. If it approaches something that it may not recognise as dangerous, a stamp of the owner's feet will cause it to stop what it is doing and run to safety.

16 ANAESTHESIA AND SURGERY

INTRODUCTION

Traditionally rabbit anaesthesia was considered a high-risk procedure, but with the advent of new anaesthetics, and a greater understanding of the rabbit patient, this view is changing. As with the anaesthesia of any species it is important to use regimes that are familiar. However, there are some important physiological factors that must be taken into consideration.

- The rabbit has a very small thoracic cavity in proportion to its body size. When the rabbit is positioned in dorsal recumbency it is important to raise the chest above the abdomen. If this is not done the weight of the abdominal contents will rest on the chest and further compromise the chest space. Rabbits also have poorly developed intercostal muscles which make expansion of the thoracic cavity difficult.
- Rabbits may be subclinically affected with *Pasteurella*, and this may influence respiration during anaesthesia.
- Rabbits are very susceptible to stress, and the catecholamines released will affect the anaesthetic, and may cause post-surgical gastric ileus. Stress should be minimised wherever possible.
- Rabbits possess atropinase which readily deactivates atropine, so atropine has no value in rabbits.
- Obese rabbits may have a large percentage of body fat, and anaesthetic dose rates should be lowered accordingly.

HOSPITALISATION

If possible, rabbits should be kept in a separate area from other animals, particularly dogs and cats which are their natural predators. The sights and smells of dogs and cats will increase stress. The rabbit area should be warm and quiet. If the rabbit is part of a pair-bond, the healthy partner should be allowed to accompany its sick companion whenever possible, even if it is just for day surgery. The sick companion will recover much faster if its partner is present, and any complications associated with re-pairing these rabbits are avoided.

Fresh greens and hay should be provided, and water given in a container to which the rabbit is accustomed.

PRE-ANAESTHETIC PREPARATION

Rabbits should not be starved before surgery. They are unable to vomit so there is no risk of aspiration of stomach contents. A period of starvation will cause hepatic lipidosis, and will delay the onset of eating after surgery. Post-anaesthetic gastric ileus is also more common.

Stress should be minimised by the administration of some premedication.

If the patient is dehydrated fluids should be given intravenously or subcutaneously before surgery. Hypoglycaemia is a potential problem in any rabbit, particularly if its appetite has been reduced, and lactated Ringer's solution or glucose–saline can be given: up to 80–100 ml can be given at one time. A sick rabbit should be stabilised as well as possible before being anaesthetised; if fluids have been given subcutaneously they will take 6–8 hours to be fully adsorbed, and if possible anaesthesia should be delayed until the rabbit is hydrated.

PREMEDICATION

The use of premedication will reduce the stress of anaesthetic induction, and will also allow the rabbit to be maintained on a lower percentage of inhalation anaesthesia. Some premedication drugs are good analgesics, and will give post-operative analgesia as well.

Acepromazine (ACP) can be given at a dose of 0.1–0.5 mg/kg by subcutaneous injection. It is not analgesic, and causes vasodilation. This facilitates subsequent intravenous injections and blood collection. ACP can be combined with buprenorphine to provide sedation and analgesia. ACP at a dose of 0.1 mg/kg and buprenorphine at a dose of 0.01 mg/kg can be combined in the same syringe and given by subcutaneous or intramuscular injection.

Butorphanol can be given at a dose of 0.1–0.5 mg/kg by subcutaneous injection. This will also provide post-operative analgesia of 3–4 hours' duration and is particularly useful for ovariohysterectomy cases.

Buprenorphine can be given at a dose of 0.01–0.05 mg/kg by subcutaneous injection. This will also provide post-anaesthetic analgesia of 6–12 hours' duration.

Diazepam can be given at a dose of 2 mg/kg by intramuscular injection.

SEDATION

Some procedures such as dental work, tear duct flushes and the lancing of abscesses can be done under sedation alone. Various drug combinations are suitable. Combinations that include either xylazine, medetomidine or butorphanol will also have an analgesic effect. The rabbit must be constantly observed as the sedation takes effect to avoid it adopting a position that could compromise its airway. Close monitoring is also important during recovery for the same reason. Most of these sedatives cause hypoxia, and the administration of oxygen via a face mask or endotracheal tube during the period of sedation is recommended.

Xylazine at a dose of 5 mg/kg and ketamine at a dose of 25–35 mg/kg can be mixed in the same syringe and given by intramuscular injection. Sedation is achieved in 5–10 minutes, and full recovery may take several hours, during which time the patient should be kept warm and turned regularly.

Ketamine at a dose of 15 mg/kg and medetomidine at a dose of 0.25 mg/kg can be mixed in the same syringe and given by intramuscular or subcutaneous injection. This combination can be reversed with atipamezole at a dose of 1 mg/kg given by intramuscular or subcutaneous injection. Recovery from ketamine and medetomidine alone may take 2 hours; if reversed with atipamezole recovery is even quicker.

Ketamine (30–40 mg/kg) and diazepam (2 mg/kg) can be given in combination by intramuscular injection.

Sedation and analgesia can be provided with the combination of ketamine (10 mg/kg), medetomidine (0.2 mg/kg) and butorphanol (0.1 mg/kg) given by intramuscular injection. This can be reversed with 1 mg/kg atipamezole by intramuscular injection without losing the analgesic effects.

Fentanyl/fluanisone (Hypnorm, Janssen Animal Health) can be given at a dose of 0.3 ml/kg by intramuscular injection in combination with diazepam (1 mg/kg) or midazolam (2 mg/kg) by intraperitoneal injection.

Surgical anaesthesia and muscle relaxation lasts for 20–40 minutes. This sedation can be partially reversed with buprenorphine (0.01–0.05 mg/kg) or butorphanol (0.1 mg/kg) by subcutaneous injection.

INHALATION ANAESTHESIA

Gaseous anaesthetics can be administered with oxygen. Nitrous oxide should not be used in the rabbit as it increases the tendency of the gastrointestinal tract to bloat.

Isoflurane is the anaesthetic of choice for rabbits. It is not as noxious as halothane and there is less of a tendency to breath hold during induction. Induction can be done with a concentration of 4%, and anaesthesia can be maintained with 1–2%. Lower concentrations are possible if the rabbit has received premedication. As 98% of the isoflurane is expelled through the lungs, recovery is rapid and no stress is placed on other organs such as the liver and kidneys.

Halothane can be used to induce anaesthesia at a concentration of 4–5% and anaesthesia can be maintained with 2%, or lower if a premedicant drug has been given. Care must be taken as halothane sensitises the myocardium to the arrhythmic effects of adrenaline (released in the stress of handling).

Induction

The procedure of induction must be as stress-free as possible. Rabbits that have been sedated will be more relaxed. Rabbits have a tendency to breath-hold if stressed, and this is accompanied by bradycardia, hypercapnia and hypoxia.

The author first trances the patient by holding it upside-down and stroking it along the bridge of the nose. When the rabbit is relaxed oxygen is introduced through a face mask. After the rabbit has breathed oxygen for 2–3 minutes the anaesthetic gas is introduced, and induction proceeds smoothly (Figure 16.1). Care should be taken not to hold the rabbit tightly around the chest during restraint.

Maintenance of anaesthesia

Anaesthesia can be maintained via a face mask, or endotracheal tube. The placing of an endotracheal tube takes experience, and after several failed

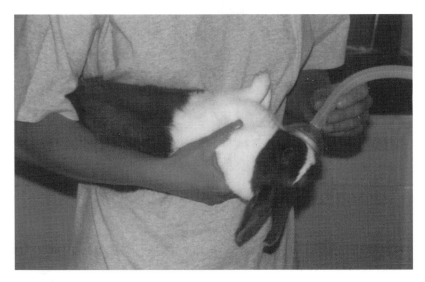

Figure 16.1   Oxygen and anaesthetic gas can be introduced through a face mask. Care is taken not to hold the rabbit tightly around the chest.

attempts a face mask should be used, as rabbits are prone to laryngeal oedema. With a good scavenging system for the waste anaesthetic gas a face mask is sufficient for short procedures.

The rabbit should be kept on a heat pad during surgery, and its temperature monitored by rectal thermometer. The rabbit's temperature can drop dramatically, particularly during abdominal surgery, and even during minor procedures rabbits have a tendency to become hypothermic.

Endotracheal intubation

Endotracheal intubation can be difficult in rabbits, particularly the smaller breeds. The shape of the rabbit's mouth makes it difficult to open it wide to visualise the back of the throat. Small rabbits require a 2 mm endotracheal tube; larger rabbits may require a 4 mm tube. Intubation can be done under direct visualisation of the larynx, or blind. Intubation is generally only possible if the rabbit is heavily sedated. Several failed attempts at intubation may cause laryngeal haemorrhage and oedema, and after three attempts a face mask should be used instead, as rabbits with traumatised airways do poorly post-operatively.

For direct visualisation the rabbit is placed in dorsal recumbency and the larynx viewed with an otoscope. The larynx can be sprayed with lignocaine to reduce the risk of laryngospasm. After visualising the larynx, an introducer is passed into the trachea (a urinary catheter can be used for this) and the otoscope removed. The endotracheal tube can the be passed over the introducer into the trachea. The rabbit may cough as the tube enters the trachea indicating its correct placement.

For intubation without visualisation of the larynx, the rabbit is held in sternal recumbency with its head stretched up. The endotracheal tube is advanced to the larynx and observed carefully. The presence of condensation in the tube, or audible breath sounds through the tube, indicate that the tube is close to the larynx. As the rabbit breathes in the tube is advanced. The continued presence of breath sounds indicates that the tube is in place. The rabbit may also cough as the tube enters the trachea.

Anaesthetic monitoring

Monitoring of the patient is important during surgery. The rectal temperature should be frequently checked as rabbits have a tendency to hypothermia. The depth of anaesthesia can be monitored by the ear pinch and hind-leg withdrawal reflex which should be just present. The foreleg withdrawal disappears later, and if this is absent the anaesthetic must be lightened. Unlike dog and cat patients, the position of the eye during anaesthesia is not significant and is not helpful in monitoring the depth of anaesthesia. Chewing is a sign of light anaesthesia, and may be associated with a rapid awakening from the anaesthesia. Heart and respiration rates should also be monitored.

POST-OPERATIVE CARE

The rabbit should be allowed to recover in a warm peaceful environment. If it is one of a pair-bond its partner should be introduced as soon as possible. Food and water should be offered, particularly tempting greens such as kale and parsley.

Sutures are best protected with light dressings. Rabbits do not tolerate Elizabethan collars well; they are unable to practice coprophagy and may become anorexic and depressed.

Post-operative analgesia should be given unless analgesia was given preoperatively, or as part of a sedative combination.

- Aspirin (100 mg/kg) orally every 12–24 hours.
- Butorphanol (0.1 mg/kg) by subcutaneous injection every 8 hours.

- Buprenorphine (0.01–0.05 mg/kg) by subcutaneous injection every 8–12 hours.
- Carprophen (1.5–2 mg/kg) given orally or by subcutaneous injection every 12–24 hours.
- Flunixin (1.1 mg/kg) by subcutaneous injection every 24 hours.
- Ketoprofen (1–3 mg/kg) by subcutaneous injection every 24 hours.
- Meloxicam (0.1–0.2 mg/kg) orally every 24 hours.

SURGICAL PROCEDURES

Descriptions of specific surgery are covered in detail in relevant places in the text. However, a few general considerations should be mentioned.

The rabbit has a great tendency to form post-surgical adhesions, particularly after abdominal surgery. It is possible that the talcum powder on sterile surgeon's gloves may trigger adhesion formation, and it is important to wear gloves without powder inside, or wash the powder off the gloves. Adhesion formation is more common with the use of chromic catgut. Although this suture material is acceptable for routine castrations and ovariohysterectomies, a synthetic absorbable suture should be chosen for more complicated abdominal surgery.

If there is concern about post-surgical adhesions, verapmil can be given by intraperitoneal injection at a dose of 0.2 mg/kg every 8 hours for nine doses.

Rabbits are very good at removing their own skin sutures. However, they do not tolerate Elizabethan collars (the standard method of preventing other companion animals from interfering with their sutures); they become depressed and are unable to practice coprophagy.

Alternatives to the simple interrupted skin suture are subcuticular sutures with a synthetic absorbable suture, a continuous close apposition (interlocking) suture with synthetic non-absorbable material, or skin staples. Skin staples are generally well tolerated; however, there is still a small risk that they could be removed, and worse, ingested by the rabbit. The author prefers the continuous interlocking suture. It is a quick and easy method of wound closure, and appears difficult for the rabbit to undo. Even if part of the suture gets bitten through, the interlocking nature of the suture means that the wound remains in apposition to allow healing to take place.

17 DRUGS AND TREATMENTS

The majority of drugs available are not licensed for use in rabbits and due care and sensible judgement must be taken when administering any treatment to rabbits.

Treatments can be given by injection or orally.

INJECTION TECHNIQUES

Small gauge needles (22–27 gauge) should be used for injections to minimise discomfort. For accurate dosing an insulin syringe may be recommended.

Subcutaneous injections are given in the scruff of the neck. This site is also suitable for the administration of subcutaneous fluids as rabbits have a large subcuticular space under the neck and shoulders.

Intramuscular injections can be given in the cranial aspect of the quadriceps muscle. Only small volumes should be administered in this way (up to 1.5 ml in a large rabbit).

Intravenous injections can be given into the cephalic or lateral saphenous veins. Care should be used if the marginal ear veins are used, as many drugs are irritant and may cause sloughing of the pinna.

Catheterisation

Intravenous catheters can be placed in the cephalic or lateral saphenous veins for the administration of fluids. In the conscious patient the cephalic vein is preferable, as it is less affected by the rabbit moving its legs. The catheter should be bandaged on well to prevent the rabbit removing it.

Intraosseous catheterisation is required for very debilitated rabbits for whom intravenous catheterisation may be impossible. Ideally this technique should be practised on some cadavers first. The femur is the most frequently used site, although catheters can be placed in the humerus or tibia. The procedure is painful and should be done under anaesthesia, or local anaesthetic. A 20–22 gauge spinal or hypodermic needle can be used; with the latter a stylet can be made using sterile surgical wire. The placement of the catheter should be done under sterile surgical conditions. The area over the head of the femur is clipped up, a small incision is made over the proximal aspect of the greater trochanter, and the needle is introduced through the trochanteric fossa into the marrow cavity. 3–5 ml of sterile saline can be injected slowly to test the patency of the catheterisation. The needle should be flushed with heparinised saline and capped. Any medication and fluids should be administered very slowly through this route. Parental antibiotics should be used while the catheter is in place, and for a few days after.

ORAL MEDICATION

Oral medication may be formulated as a liquid or tablets. Liquids can be easily syringed into the mouth, or, where appropriate added to the drinking water. Tablets can be mixed with a favourite food such as banana, or mixed with strawberry jam.

Debilitated rabbits that may have a nasogastric tube in place can be given liquid medication through this route (see Chapter 9).

DRUG TREATMENTS AND DOSE RATES

Antibiotics

Whenever possible antibiotic use should be based on the results of bacterial culture and sensitivity. If this is not possible, a broad spectrum antibiotic should be chosen. Narrow spectrum antibiotics, especially those with an action on Gram-positive organisms, have the potential to cause a fatal enterotoxaemia. Rabbits should be protected from this consequence by the concurrent use of a probiotic, and by ensuring that they are on a good quality high fibre (hay) diet.

The safest antibiotics are enrofloxacin and trimethoprim–sulpha combinations. In some circumstances such as abscesses or *Pasteurella* infection, antibiosis may be required for weeks or months, and both of these antibiotics are safe for long term use.

Narrow spectrum antibiotics such as cephaloridine, cephalexin and penicillin should only be used if specifically indicated, and then administered by injection only.

Cephalexin
Ceporex Injection (Schering-Plough Animal Health)

Cephalexin is a narrow spectrum antibiotic, and should only be used in cases where it is specifically indicated, and then by subcutaneous injection alone.

Dose: 20 mg/kg once daily. Ceporex injection contains 180 mg/ml cephalexin and this approximates to a dose of 0.11 ml/kg.

Enrofloxacin
Baytril (Bayer plc)

Dose: 5–10 mg/kg daily, or twice daily in severe infections. 10 mg/kg once daily is sufficient in most cases and once daily dosing is less stressful for the patient. The 2.5% injection contains 25 mg/ml enrofloxacin and can be given by subcutaneous injection. Repeated injections may cause sterile abscesses at the injection site, and the injection can be irritant resulting in self-trauma, so long term medication should be oral.

The 2.5% oral solution is the most useful for oral dosing; this also contains 25 mg/ml enrofloxacin and can be given neat at a dose of 0.4 ml/kg daily, or diluted 1:1 with blackcurrant syrup to increase its palatability and given at a dose of 0.8 ml/kg daily. Alternatively the 2.5% oral solution can be diluted in the drinking water at a rate of 1 ml:250 ml to produce a concentration of 100 mg/litre.

Baytril is a good broad spectrum antibiotic, and is safe for long term use. Its use should be avoided in very young rabbits as it may cause swollen joints.

Metronidazole
Flagyl-S suspension (May and Baker Ltd.)

This may be useful in cases of enterotoxaemia to prevent clostridial multiplication.

Dose: 20–30 mg/kg orally twice a day. The suspension contains 40 mg/ ml metronidazole, and this approximates to a dose of 0.5 ml/kg twice daily.

Neomycin
Neobiotic pump (Upjohn Ltd.)

Dose: This can be used in cases of enteritis at a dose of 30 mg/kg orally twice a day. The solution contains 50 mg/ml neomycin, and this approximates to a dose of 0.6 ml/kg twice daily.

Oxytetracycline
Engemycin 5% (Intervet UK Ltd.)

This formulation is useful for the long-term treatment of abscesses that are not amenable to complete incision.

Dose: 30 mg/kg by subcutaneous injection every third day. This formulation contains 50 mg/ml, which approximates to a dose of 0.6 ml/kg.

Terramycin soluble powder 5.5% (Pfizer Ltd.)

This drug is useful in Tyzzers disease.

Dose: Terramycin can be used in the drinking water at a concentration of 125 mg/litre for up to a month. One level scoop of powder (4 g) contains approximately 200 mg of oxytetracycline, and can be dissolved in 1.6 litres of water to achieve this concentration.

A higher dose of 250 mg/litre can be used over the period of weaning to prevent weaning enteritis or *Pasteurella* infection.

Penicillin
Ampicillin: Amfipen (Intervet UK Ltd.)

Dose: 25 mg/kg once daily by intramuscular or subcutaneous injection. Amfipen 15% contains 150 mg/ml ampicillin, and this gives a dose of 0.16 ml/kg daily.

Penicillin should only be used against *Treponema* infections, or in *Pasteurella* infections that do not respond to other antibiotics. The rabbit must be on a good high fibre diet and probiotic.

Procaine penicillin: Penillin (Vétquinol UK Ltd.)

Dose: Penillin contains 300 mg (300 000 iu)/ml of procaine penicillin. For *Treponema* infections the dose is 40 000 iu/kg (0.13 ml/kg) daily for 7 days by intramuscular injection. Alternatively a dose of 80 000 iu/kg (0.26 ml/kg) can be given once a week by intramuscular injection.

Duplocillin LA (Intervet UK Ltd.)

Dose: Duplocillin contains 150 mg/ml procaine penicillin and 112.5 mg/ ml benzathine penicillin. It can be given weekly by intramuscular injection at a dose of 0.1 ml/kg.

Sulpha drugs

These drugs are particularly useful against coccidiosis.

Sulphadimidine
Intradine (Norbrook Laboratories Ltd.)

Dose: Intradine contains 33% w/v sulphadimidine and can be given in the drinking water at a concentration of 0.2%. To achieve this concentration 1 ml of sulphamezathine 33% can be diluted in 150 ml water. This can be given as three 3 day courses, with two 2 day intervals in between.

Trimethoprim–sulpha
Borgal (Hoechst Roussel Vet Ltd.)

Dose: The dose is based on the total trimethroprim and sulpha content of the drug and is 30 mg/kg twice daily by injection or orally.

  Borgal 7.5% solution contains 62.5 mg/ml sulfadoxine and 12.5 mg/ml trimethoprim; therefore a total of 75 mg/ml. The dose by injection is 0.4 ml/kg twice daily.

Septrin Paediatric Suspension (Glaxo/Wellcome)

Dose: This contains 8 mg/ml trimethoprim and 40 mg/ml sulpha-methoxazole; therefore a total of 48 mg/ml. The oral dose is 0.6 ml/kg twice daily. This antibiotic is banana flavoured and readily accepted by the rabbit.

Probiotics

Probiotics contain live bacteria, and are useful in times of stress, illness and antibiotic usage. The live bacteria are in an encapsulated form so that they are able to survive passage through the low pH of the stomach and enter the caecum. They do not colonise the caecum, but in large numbers are able to provide competition against more harmful bacteria, and hence have a protective effect on the caecal flora and help stabilise gut activity.

Avipro (VetArk Health)

This is a water soluble probiotic containing *Lactobacillus acidophilus*, *Enterococcus faecium*, *Saccharomyces* and electrolytes. This can be diluted 5 g into 200 ml water, or if syringe feeding a pinch can be added to every feed.

Analgesics

Aspirin

Dose: 100 mg/kg orally, every 12–24 hours. Tablets can be crushed and given orally. A total dose of 75–150 mg is often sufficient for an average rabbit.

Buprenorphine
Vetergesic (Animalcare Ltd.)

Dose: 0.01–0.05 mg/kg by subcutaneous injection. Analgesia lasts 6–12 hours. If given pre-operatively it will reduce the concentration of isoflurane required for maintenance of anaesthesia. Vetergesic contains 0.3 mg/ml buprenorphine and this approximates to a dose of 0.03–0.16 ml/kg.

Butorphanol
Torbugesic (Fort Dodge Animal Health)

Dose: 0.1–0.5 mg/kg by subcutaneous injection. Analgesia lasts 3–4 hours. If given pre-operatively it will reduce the concentration of isoflurane required for maintenance of anaesthesia. Torbugesic contains 10 mg/ml of butorphanol and this approximates to a dose of 0.01–0.05 ml/kg. An insulin syringe is recommended for accurate dosing.

Carprofen
Rimadyl (Pfizer Animal Health Ltd.)

Dose: 1.5–2 mg/kg orally twice daily: Rimadyl 20 tablets contain 20 mg of carprofen and can be used for this.

The injection can be given daily at a dose of 2 mg/kg subcutaneously and will give approximately 12 hours' analgesia. It can be given pre-operatively. The injection contains 50 mg/ml carprofen and this approximates to a injectable dose of 0.04 ml/kg.

Flunixine
Finadyne Injection for Dogs (Schering-Plough Animal Health)

Dose: 1.1 mg/kg by subcutaneous injection.

The injection contains 10 mg/ml flunixine and this approximates to a dose of 0.11 ml/kg.

An oral solution can be given twice daily at a dose of 1.1 mg/kg. The injectable form can be mixed 1:4 with blackcurrant syrup to give a concentration of 2 mg/ml flunixine and given orally at a dose of 0.5 ml/kg twice daily.

For long term dosing this drug can be given every other day, or 5 days in succession and then 2 days off.

Ketoprofen
Ketofen 1% (Merial Animal Health Ltd.)

Dose: 1 mg/kg by intramuscular injection once daily. The 1% injectable solution contains 10 mg/kg ketoprofen and this approximates to a dose of 0.1 ml/kg.

Meloxicam
Metacam Oral Suspension (Boehringer Ingelheim Ltd.)

Dose: 0.1–0.2 mg/kg orally once a day. The oral suspension contains 1.5 mg/ml meloxicam. One drop contains 0.1 mg meloxicam, and this approximates to a dose of 1–2 drops per kilogram orally.

Miscellaneous treatments

Cisapride
Prepulsid (Janssen-Cilag)

This is a motility drug with a different mode of action to metoclopramide, and both drugs can be given simultaneously.

Dose: 0.5–1 mg/kg orally every 8–24 hours. The tablets contain 10 mg cisapride and an average 2.5 kg rabbit can be given one-quarter of a tablet three times a day.

Corticosteroids

These should not be used for long term treatment as their immunosuppressive action may precipitate latent *Pasteurella* infections. Long term use may also precipitate diabetes. The exceptions are cases of atopy or auto-immune disease. Corticosteroids are, however, very useful for the immediate treatment of shock, intervertebral disc protrusion, and head-tilt.

Dexamethasone
Dexadreson (Intervet UK Ltd.)

Dose: This contains 2 mg/ml dexamethasone and can be given at a dose of 0.5–2 mg/kg (equivalent to 0.25–1 ml/kg) by intravenous, intramuscular or subcutaneous injection. A 'shock' dose is 2 mg/kg.

Prednisolone

Dose: This can be used for long-term management of atopy or auto-immune disease at a dose of 0.5–2 mg/kg daily.

Fenbendazole
Panacur (Hoechst Roussel Vet Ltd.)

This is an anthelmintic, useful against roundworms and pinworms.

Dose: 10–20 mg/kg orally. The 2.5% suspension contains 25 mg/ml of fenbendazole, and this approximates to a dose of 0.4 ml/kg given orally. The treatment can be repeated after 14 days.

Frusemide
Frusecare tablets 40 mg (Animalcare Ltd.)

This is a diuretic and can be used in cases of congestive heart failure.

Dose: 2–5 mg/kg orally twice a day. A 2.5 kg rabbit can be given one-quarter of a tablet twice a day.

Ivermectin
Ivomec Injection for Sheep (Merial Animal Health Ltd.)

This is an antiparasitic drug and can be used to control ectoparasites. It is also effective against roundworms.

Dose: 0.4 mg/kg by subcutaneous injection. The injectable form contains 1% w/v ivermectin and this approximates to a dose of 0.04 ml/kg. The treatment should be repeated fortnightly for control of most ectoparasites, and weekly for control of *Demodex*. A single dose is useful in the treatment of 'flystrike'. It can also be made up with water at a concentration of 5 mg/l (0.5 ml in 1 litre of water) to use as a spray when treating flystrike. A single injection is sufficient for control of roundworm. A 1% ivermectin 'spot-on' preparation is available for pigeons, and this can be used to control *Cheyletiella*. A single drop is applied to the skin behind the ear and repeated fortnightly.

Metoclopramide
Emequell (Pfizer Ltd.)

Metoclopramide restores normal co-ordination and tone to the upper digestive tract, and is useful for promoting gastrointestinal motility in cases of gastric ileus or stasis.

Dose: 0.2–1 mg/kg up to four times a day, orally or by subcutaneous or intramuscular injection. Emequell injection contains 5 mg/ml metoclopramide and this approximates to a dose of 0.1 ml/kg. Emequell tablets contain 10 mg metoclopramide and a 2.5 kg rabbit can be given one-quarter of a tablet 3–4 times daily.

Vitamin B$_{12}$

Multivit B$_{12}$ injection (C-Vet Veterinary Products)

Dose: 20–50 µg/kg. The injection contains 250 µg/ml and a dose of 0.2 ml/kg can be given.

18 ZOONOTIC ASPECTS

Very few zoonotic diseases have been documented in rabbits. People with a healthy immune system have a resistance to most diseases; however, if they are immunocompromised through concurrent disease, if they are young, or if they are taking immunosuppressive drugs, the risks of contracting a zoonotic disease are higher. One common hazard for owners is the consequence of a bite or scratch, which may become infected, and some owners may develop respiratory allergies to the rabbit's fur, urinary proteins or bedding.

CHEYLETIELLA

This is the most frequently recorded zoonosis; this mite causes a transient pruritic rash in humans. It is spread by direct contact with the rabbit, and from its contaminated bedding. The mite is easily identifiable and the rabbit can be treated with ivermectin. All the bedding should be changed and the environment treated with an insecticide. Pet dogs that come in contact with the rabbit should be examined and treated as necessary, as they can be affected by *Cheyletiella* as well.

FLEAS

Rabbits can harbour fleas. This may become increasingly common as house rabbits mix with other pets such as dogs and cats that may carry fleas. The rabbit, other household pets and the environment should be treated accordingly.

PSOROPTES

The rabbit ear mite rarely infects humans. Both the rabbit and the environment should be treated, as the mite can survive successfully off the rabbit for several weeks.

TRICHOPHYTON

Ringworm is the second most common zoonosis, and can also affect other in-contact pets if the rabbit is a house rabbit. Children are particularly at risk of infection. Gloves should be worn whilst treating the rabbit to avoid infection. Transmission of *Trichophyton* can also be from human to rabbit.

PASTEURELLA

Bites or scratches inflicted by the rabbit may become infected, particularly if the rabbit is harbouring *Pasteurella*. Any bite or cut should be immediately washed in a disinfectant solution. Rabbits can be serologically tested and this should be recommended, particularly if the owner is immuno-compromised.

Rarely, *Pasteurella* can cause a dermatitis in humans, also very rarely arthritis, meningitis, peritonitis, pneumonia and septicaemia.

ENTERIC BACTERIA

Rabbits can become infected with *Salmonella*, *Campylobacter*, and enteropathogenic *Escherichia coli*. The sources of infection for rabbit and human are contaminated unwashed vegetables and food. Although the zoonotic potential is small, if there is an immunocompromised person in the household it is advisable occasionally to culture fresh faeces to screen for enteric pathogens.

Yersinia pseudotuberculosis can also affect humans, but infections are extremely rare.

ENCEPHALITOZOONOSIS

Rabbits are the principal hosts of this protozoal parasite, but *Encephalitozoon cuniculi* has been reported in other rodents (mice, hamsters, guinea pigs and rats) and mammals (dogs, cats and squirrel monkeys). Cases of disseminated *E. cuniculi* have recently been reported in AIDS patients. It is possible that other immunosuppressed humans, such as those on chemotherapy or immunosuppressive drugs may be at risk, although as yet there is no documented evidence of a direct transfer of infection from rabbit to human. Clinical signs in humans include chronic diarrhoea, hepatitis, pneumonitis, renal symptoms, corneal infection and sinusitis.

Rabbits that may come into contact with immunosuppressed patients should be serologically tested, and strict sanitation must be practised, because the organism is spread in the urine.

TULARAEMIA

This is a potentially zoonotic disease in wild rabbits, and although it has not yet been identified in pet rabbits, where rabbits are housed outdoors in areas where wild rabbits exist, there is potential for it to be spread from the wild population. Tularaemia is caused by the bacterium *Francisella tularensis* and it is spread by biting insects, mosquitos and ticks. It causes a fatal septicaemia in rodents, rabbits and some birds (pheasants and quail). It is prevalent in southern central United States.

Francisella tularensis is harboured in the tissues, blood and faeces of an infected rabbit, and humans can be infected through skin lesions, or by tick bites. For this reason gloves should be worn when handling potentially infective material.

Clinical signs of human tularaemia are cutaneous lesions, septicaemia and meningitis.

REFERENCES AND FURTHER READING

Ackerman, S. and Deeb, B. (1998). Head tilt: causes and treatment. *American House Rabbit Journal* (http://www.rabbit.org/journal/3-8/head-tilt.html).

Besch-Williford, C. (1997). *Encephalitozoon cuniculi:* an update on epidemiology, diagnosis and control of the disease. In: *Rabbit Medicine and Procedures for Practitioners*. Program and abstracts from American House Rabbit Society Veterinary Conference, Berkeley, CA, pp. 47–50.

Bower, J. and Bowers, C. (1998). *Top to Tail, A Grown-up's Guide to Rabbit Care*. Petplan, Middlesex.

Brown, S. (1993). Anorectic rabbit protocol. *Rabbit Health News*, **9**, 3–4.

Brown, S. (1994). Rabbit GI physiology and diet. *Rabbit Health News*, **11**, 3–5.

Brown, S.A. (1998a). Rabbit urinary tract disease. *Notes for BSAVA Conference*, Birmingham, UK, pp. 19–20.

Brown, S.A. (1998b). Gastrointestinal physiology and disease in the domestic pet rabbit. *Rabbit Healthcare*, **1**(3), 1–6.

Cheeke, P.R. (1987). *Rabbit Feeding and Nutrition*. Academic Press, Orlando.

Clipshon, C. (1993). Allergies. *Rabbit Health News*, **9**, 2.

Cutler, S.L. (1998). Ectopic *Psoroptes cuniculi* infestation in a pet rabbit. *Journal of Small Animal Practice*, **39**, 86–87.

Divers, S.J. (1997). Incisor malocclusion in the rabbit. *Veterinary Times*, February, 12–15.

Flecknell, P. (1998). Developments in the veterinary care of rabbits and rodents. *In Practice*, **20**, 286–295.

Fuller, H.E., Lucas, M.H. and Gibbens, J.C. (1993) Rabbit haemorrhagic disease in the United Kingdom. *Veterinary Record*, **133**, 611–613.

Harcourt-Brown, F. (1996). Calcium deficiency, diet and dental disease in pet rabbits. *Veterinary Record*, **139**, 567–571.

Harcourt-Brown, F. (1997). Diagnosis, treatment and prognosis of dental disease in pet rabbits. *In Practice*, **18**, 407–421.

Harcourt-Brown, F. (1999). Pet rabbits: some common clinical problems. *Waltham Focus*, **8**(4), 6–13.

Harkness, J. (1994). Calcium in rabbits. *Rabbit Health News*, **11**, 7–8.

Harkness, J.E. and Wagner, J.E. (1989). *The Biology and Medicine of Rabbits and Rodents*. Lea and Febiger, Philadelphia.

Harriman, M. (1995). *House Rabbit Handbook*. Drollery Press, Alameda.

Harvey, C. (1997). Rabbits physical exam and differential diagnoses. In: *Rabbit Medicine and Procedures for Practitioners*. Program and abstracts from American House Rabbit Society Veterinary Conference, Berkeley, CA, pp. 7–14.

Hillyer, E.V. and Quesenberry, K.E. (1997). *Ferrets, Rabbits and Rodents. Clinical Medicine and Surgery*. W.B. Saunders, Philadelphia.

Hillyer, E.V. (1994). Pet rabbits. *Veterinary Clinics of North America*, **24**(1), 25–65.

Jenkins, J.R. (1997). Rabbit dentistry. In: *Rabbit Medicine and Procedures for Practitioners*. Program and abstracts from American House Rabbit Society Veterinary Conference, Berkeley, CA, pp. 35–38.

Jenkins, J.R. and Brown, S.A. (1993). *A Practitioner's Guide to Rabbits and Ferrets*. American Animal Hospital Association, Colorado.

Johnson-Delaney, C. (1994). Potential zoonoses from pet rabbits. *Rabbit Health News*, **12**, 1–3.

Kestenman, S. (1995). Bladder calculi and sludgy bladder. *Rabbit Health News*, **13**, 3–4.

Kirwan, A.P., Middleton, B. and McGarry, J.W. (1998). Diagnosis and prevalence of *Leporacarus gibbus* in the fur of domestic rabbits in the UK. *Veterinary Record*, **142**, 20–21.

Laber-Laird, K., Swindle, M.M. and Flecknell, P. (1996). *Rodent and Rabbit Medicine*. Pergamon Press, Oxford.

McBride, A. (1988). *Rabbits and Hares*. Whittet Books, London.

McBride, A. (1998) *Why Does My Rabbit?* Souvenir Press, London.

Malley, A.D. (1994). The pet rabbit in companion animal practice. 1. A clinician's approach to the pet rabbit. *Irish Veterinary Journal*, **47**, 9–15.

Malley, A.D. (1995a). Dental disorders of rodents and lagamorphs. *Notes for BSAVA Continuing Education Course*, Oxford.

Malley, A.D. (1995b). Some diseases of the pet rabbit. *Notes for BSAVA Continuing Education Course*, Oxford.

Morrell, J.M. (1989). Hydrometra in the rabbit. *Veterinary Record*, **125**, 325.

Overman, L. (1994). *Diseases of Domestic Rabbits*. Blackwell Science, Oxford.

Sandford, J.C. (1996). *The Domestic Rabbit*. Blackwell Science, Oxford.

Silverman, S. (1998). Radiology of pet rabbits – an overview. *Rabbit Healthcare*, **1**(3), 9–10.

Whittaker, D. (1990). Pasteurellosis in the laboratory rabbit: a review. In: *The Veterinary Annual*. Blackwell Science, Oxford.

Wiseman, J. (1987). *Feeding of Non-Ruminant Livestock*. Butterworths, London.

A source of useful information is *Rabbit Health News*, 13 issues of which were published from 1990 to 1995 by the American House Rabbit Society, PO Box 3242, Redmond, WA, USA. The editors were S. Ackerman and M. Harriman, and some of the main authors were Susan Brown, Robert C. Clipsham, Barbara Deeb, John Harkness, Jeffrey Jenkins, S. Kestenman, Diane Mitchell and Lisa V. Pfeifer.

INDEX